LET ME HELP

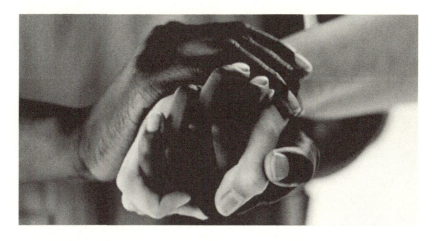

The Best Decisions Begin With Kindness

DAVID TROCK, MD

DEDICATION

This book is dedicated to Sunchita & Cyril DeGrasse Tyson for their enduring legacy of kindness, fairness, and reason.

"*Wherever there is a human being, there is an opportunity for kindness.*"

-Seneca

"*Let me help.* A hundred years or so from now, a famous novelist will write a classic using that theme. He'll recommend those three words even over *I love you.*"

-James T. Kirk (to Edith Keeler, Earth 1930)

* Star Trek quote courtesy of CBS Studios

TABLE OF CONTENTS

PART 1

Let Me Help

For several years I served as an attending at a Veterans Hospital arthritis clinic where a friendly old war vet named Frank Bering received care for rheumatoid arthritis. His fingers were too twisted to shake hands normally so he greeted his buddies with a pat on the arm. He had a crooked walking stick with a duck's head carved at the top and bulky orthopedic shoes that fastened with Velcro ties. Rain or shine, he arrived with a limp and a smile.

"How are you doing there, Frank?" the other vets would say, to which he'd respond with a cheerful "Happy to be alive another day." There was just no getting him down. Most people would have grumbled in Frank's shoes, but he refused to complain; instead, he told jokes and stories that lifted the spirits of those around him. Dr. Bob Gifford ran the arthritis clinic and shared a wink whenever old Frank shuffled in, as if tapping into his energy. The other patients noticed it too; it seemed that Frank had a gift of getting people to briefly set aside their own problems.

Then one day Frank Bering stopped coming to the clinic. We weren't sure if he had died or moved away, or if he'd taken his own life which happens sometimes to men in his situation, but we talked about him as if he were still alive. The friendly old war veteran with crippling arthritis was clearly missed.

On a whim, I called his home phone number to express my concern, if not my condolences, and it turned out that Frank Bering had indeed died—but my other assumptions about him were entirely wrong. His widow handed the phone to his grown daughter who was amused by my kind remembrances.

"Nice guy?" she said. "Are we talking about the same man? Dad was a mean drunk half the time and not much better when he was sober. He was always miserable and spent the whole day watching TV alone. The only thing that made him happy was going to the damn clinic."

I listened to his daughter's rant and wondered who is the real Frank Bering? He seemed like the sweetest guy around. When she had finally run out of steam, I wished her well and hung up thinking maybe I shouldn't have called.

At the next clinic, Dr. Gifford and I stepped into the waiting area to share the news that Frank had passed away, nothing more. The vets bowed their heads and saluted his memory by telling his favorite jokes and stories, and within minutes their smiles were replaced by laughter. They passed around a photo of his crazy walking stick with the duck's head, and for the time being it seemed like their problems had drifted far away.

Let me help

Caring for patients requires a well of concern for those in need and a helping hand at the ready, which means setting aside your own issues in order to ask the question, "What can I do for you?" Once this question is asked, the rest flows more easily. The general sentiment and the title of this book give patients what they are looking for: a chance to be well, to be reassured, or at least find answers. And it feels good to help, even if the best you can do is try. The gratification on both sides is worth the time and effort that goes into training, which is something to remember if you're just getting started.

One of the key themes of this book is *kindness*, which is at odds with adversity and illness, and those in the helping professions wage a daily battle. Sometimes we win and sometimes we lose, but we always show up.

The rewards of kindness are oddly reciprocal; for example, providers who are consistently kind to patients are thought of as better *clinicians*. This "halo effect" is evident in the evaluations given to doctors, nurses, PA's, and medical students. It's a reward for being nice. It helps caregivers maintain a good reputation in the community. Conversely, those whose demeanors are terse, brusque, impatient, or intolerant are perceived as less-effective caregivers, regardless of their intelligence or actual clinical outcomes. This is also seen in evaluations posted on social media and is typically an unspoken sentiment among colleagues.

When doctors and nurses are asked to make referrals to other medical specialists their choices are based on clinical skill, availability, and *kindness*. If a patient of mine was mistreated by an overworked or unhappy caregiver, I would hear about it at some point and I'd be reluctant to make another referral. It goes without saying that the attitudes we put forth, even when we think nobody is looking, do not go unnoticed. Our colleagues and patients watch everything we say and do, and that's a good thing.

In the healthcare community, word spreads quickly. Each medical office has a *personality* of its own that is judged by reasonable people who expect to be treated with kindness and respect, not only as patients but *paying customers*, with quality service and efficiency.

Like most businesses, the atmosphere of a medical office or hospital ward begins at the top, and when employees and staff are treated well by their supervisors, the patients are among the first to benefit. The long-term results are evident: better job satisfaction and better clinical results.

What is kindness?

Kindness is an agreeable way of treating others. It is not quite a sentiment or an emotion but a form of *behavior,* such as holding a door open for the next person or comforting a frightened patient. Kindness is shown by volunteering at a food drive, mowing the lawn of a sick neighbor, or supporting a nearby pet shelter. The extremes of kindness extend to donating a kidney or adopting a special needs child, but how many are willing to make such a personal sacrifice? Can those who never reach that level of service to humanity claim to be truly kind? The answer is yes, of course.

Surveys show that 90% of people think of *themselves* as kind, yet only 50% believe that *others* are kind. Think about that for a moment. Like the 90% of motorists in surveys who consider themselves "above-average drivers" (which is mathematically difficult) it appears that we are similarly biased when we think of ourselves as kind. To be fair, some people are kinder than others, and perhaps 90% of people are kind based on *their own* assessment (even if others may not agree). So, what does it all mean, and what have we learned from recent events in healthcare?

At the onset of the COVID-19 pandemic, frontline healthcare workers were faced with the uncertain danger of a new lethal virus. Despite wearing masks, gowns and gloves, many were infected by the very people whose lives they were trying to save. Month after month they reported for long shifts despite the risk to themselves and their loved ones. Some didn't make it. Nearly 100,000 healthcare workers died during the first 18 months of the pandemic and others remained sick with post-COVID symptoms. The few times I had to suit up for consultation in the Intensive Care Unit were unsettling and uncomfortable, but it was nothing compared to those who remained in protective gear all day.

We talk about kindness and courage, but what is the proper word for the efforts made by healthcare workers during the surge of HIV/AIDS in the early 1980's or the Ebola crisis in 2015, or the ongoing risks taken by *Doctors Without Borders* in war-torn, impoverished nations? Kindness is just the tip of the iceberg.

Unlike *compassion*, which is a heightened sensitivity to the distress of others and a desire to alleviate their suffering, *kindness* is a form of *behavior*, a skill that can be *learned*. Kindness is a *choice*. By contrast, compassion (like empathy) is largely *inherent*—you either have it or you don't—which may explain why compassion is not easily taught. *Kindness can be taught.*

Not to be confused with *altruism* (giving up something despite a risk or cost to one's self, such as sharing resources in the face of scarcity) kindness can be given with nothing lost. It may overlap with altruism: for example, donating money to charity, although cynics would argue that for certain wealthy individuals a charitable tax deduction is self-serving and therefore not entirely altruistic. Aristotle defined kindness as *"helpfulness towards someone in need, not in return for anything, nor for the advantage of the helper himself, but for the person helped,"* which sounds a lot like altruism.

Ayn Rand took a more rigid stance in "The Virtue of Selfishness" claiming that helping others in need *is not* the ideal of morality; rather, she warned that *too much effort* toward selfless altruism can lead to stress, burnout, and poor mental health. This is relevant since *burnout* is so prevalent in healthcare today. In Rand's objectivist world, acting only *in your own best interest* is the noblest activity—and herein lies the dilemma: are kindness and altruism one in the same, and *is it possible to serve others while also serving your own best interest?* I believe the answer is yes, and the field of healthcare represents this paradigm better than any other.

Where does kindness begin?

Kindness is one of the first things we learn, before speech or walking. An infant treated with kindness knows little else. The opposite is true as well, which underscores the impact of abuse or neglect. A two-year old toddler may not instinctively share a toy or a snack, but by kindergarten the impulse begins to shift toward sharing. By then most children learn that kindness is a reciprocal social behavior that is rewarded.

If proper limits are set with good role models around, school-age children begin to learn *frustration tolerance,* which helps later in life so that, despite the urge to scream if an airline loses your luggage or a computer suddenly deletes an important document, you know that anger will not solve the problem. We learn these lessons over and over, yet for all our days on earth we need to be *reminded.* That's because kindness and tolerance are *skills* that must be rehearsed.

The ritual of kindness, like brushing your teeth, must be routinely practiced. Show me a member of the clergy who hasn't recited the same sermon year after year—yet the same audience shows up to listen as if they're hearing it for the first time. It's the same thing with any football coach or physical therapist; their words of encouragement are repeated endlessly because people have short memories, a reminder that kindness to others is not only helpful but teachable.

Eventually, one's best intentions, shaped by events good and bad, emerge later in life as a *calling to serve*. From there we learn to reassure patients when they're afraid, listen to their worries, explain instructions, offer patience with a knowing smile, and carry on when we're dragged down by the inertia of the day. We endure despite the capricious trajectory of illnesses that are briefly conquered like the laughing odds of a casino. But we stand firm and plow through, because sick patients need us whether we're having a good day or not. It's a ritual that pulls us out of bed each morning.

With experience we learn that acts of kindness are often unexpected but are always welcome. Those who witness a kind gesture are *inspired* to do the same, and the cycle continues.

*

True story. A forty-year-old woman named Maria Santos sat on my exam table and braced herself for bad news. The test results had arrived and she was understandably worried. Our young intern was Hindu, the rotating medical student was Muslim, and my nurse was Jewish; they stood by quietly as Maria raised a hand to the crucifix around her neck. I scrolled through the data once more to be sure and told her the good news: the scans were negative, there was no evidence of cancer.

Maria gasped in relief and covered her face with both hands. After a quick moment to gather herself, she allowed hugs all around.

I felt lucky to be in that room, to live in a country where people of different ethnicities, culinary tastes, and belief systems work together, live among each other, even fall in love—and caregivers are at the center at all of it; we are there from birth to death and bear witness to everything in-between. Modern healthcare has extended the lives of people with cancer, infection, autoimmune disease, and heart disease, and the role of good bedside manner cannot be underestimated.

Patient satisfaction surveys have repeatedly shown that doctors and nurses who practice kindness make *better* providers. In fact, *teaching* kindness has been introduced into the core curriculum of modern medical training facilities: it's a humanities program called *The Healer's Art* offered to first-year students at hundreds of *Medical and Nursing Schools.* Founded by Rachel Remen, MD in 1991, *The Healer's Art lectures* foster a young caregiver's humanity and professional satisfaction in the face of heightened stress, frustration, and scrutiny. In so doing, the nascent attributes of kindness are reinvigorated and reinforced, along with case studies and hearty advice. Dr. Remen's program adds vital perspective to all who care for patients, helps to reduce job burnout, and promotes a satisfying, personal experience for both provider and patient.

Actually, much of what we learn about kindness in healthcare is *re-learned.* We enter the field as idealistic with a calling to help until an unforgiving system picks away at our romantic notions—we become tired and jaded with a dose of reality that hits hard—then gradually, with experience and confidence we find our way back to the original calling. In time, with maturity we *learn to be kind all over again.* It's how the field of healthcare creates durable caregivers, by testing and challenging us until we are ready to take a sick patient by the hand.

A pragmatist might view kindness as a useful skill that is cultivated in daily life, like having good manners (which are also learned) whereas a cynic might suggest that caregivers, like those in any service industry, should treat customers with kindness because it's what they're paid to do. These skewed opinions raise the question: is it more important for a caregiver to genuinely *be* kind than to merely *act* kind? The answer is yes, although providing kindness in the practice of medicine does not necessarily distinguish one from the other. In either case, an atmosphere of kindness results in a happier clinical staff, improved job performance, better patient compliance, and better clinical outcomes. These findings are known to experienced caregivers, though it helps to be reminded on a regular basis.

Whether you are a nurse's aide providing a sponge bath, a phlebotomist reassuring a terrified child, or a social worker preparing a discharge plan for an isolated senior, you've learned by doing. We all learn by repetition and doing, and somewhere along the way, with a little luck, we discover that being kind is nothing without the people who need our kindness. We owe them everything.

An excellent reference for caregivers is *"Compassionomics"* by Stephen Trzeciak and Anthony Mazzarelli, available in hard copy or audio-book. The authors warn that we are in the midst of a *compassion crisis* in which providers have been paying less personal attention to patients and more on their computer screens. *Compassionomics* takes a look at the available research that shows the evidence-based results of providing compassion in the clinical setting with clear benefits for patients (better lab results, improved compliance and overall survival) and measurable rewards for caregivers, too (improved career satisfaction and a happier life) when compassion is demonstrated in medicine. These attributes are reviewed in detail and serve as a reminder of why people choose a career in healthcare.

"Otherness"

A common scourge that has plagued mankind since the very beginning has been the mistreatment of newcomers, immigrants, minorities, the disabled, the underprivileged, and those who are different in any way—*the others*. It's an unflattering aspect of the human condition that is seen widely in the animal kingdom, and we are no better. Territorial suspicion, fear and ignorance are just some of the reasons that newcomers and outliers are shunned. One would think the medical arena would be immune from inconsequential superficial differences, but we are dealing with human behavior.

There is no better time to break down barriers and achieve a good rapport than during an initial encounter. When we put our best foot forward it benefits not only those who depend on us, but *all of us*. If there happens to be a racial or cultural difference between patient and caregiver, there is yet another opportunity to shine. Do this several times per day, extrapolate that over the course of a career, and you will make an important difference in the lives of many people.

"You should invite some to your table because they are deserving, and others because they may come to deserve it."

-Seneca

The Stoic philosopher Lucius Seneca uttered the above words two thousand years ago as a way of recognizing *potential* in those who have been overlooked by giving them a *chance*. His opinion is supported in today's healthcare industry where tolerance is respected and disdain for bigotry is paramount. Helping others must include *everyone* regardless of race, religion, gender, or financial status. In this way, the practice of medicine is not only about wellness but an exercise in becoming a better person.

Good caregivers know that serving the culturally disenfranchised is an essential form of kindness. Those who rush to detect the most superficial differences of others and judge them accordingly are unwilling to accept that we are all more alike than different. They make dangerous assumptions based on physical appearance, racial difference, or troubled circumstances, as if to say *that could never be me*, rather than thinking *that could easily be me.*

It sounds like empathy but it's simpler than that. Kindness is a declaration that *we are all the same.* Even our troubles are the same. If an unkempt morbidly obese woman takes the seat next to you on a train, you may feel offput in some way, but probably not as much as she feels about herself—and it would be easy to move aside or choose a different seat—but if you offer a kind word instead or ask her about the book she's reading, she may surprise you.

In the field of medicine, kindness happens one patient at a time. A Nurse Practitioner who swabs a raw strep throat and prescribes amoxicillin knows from experience that adding a comforting word takes minimal effort and has many rewards. The accumulation of kind gestures grows in time to something substantial like a meaningful life. A career in healthcare offers exactly that.

Moral ambiguity – when kindness is questioned

A quality surgeon's questionable history of drinking. Not telling an elderly woman with dementia about her terminal illness (per her family's wishes). Providing quality care to an abusive husband or a blatant bigot. Should a provider confess or apologize to a patient if a medical mistake was made? The answers to these moral quandaries may seem obvious at first, but they are all subject to debate.

One might think we should have mastered these issues long ago since moral clarity has been examined for generations, yet we remain uncertain. The biggest controversies of the day (abortion, gun control, etc.) get most of the headlines, yet we are still far from a consensus. Perhaps with civility there will be more fertile ground for discussion and answers will be found, but so far there is mostly political noise and little agreement.

In healthcare, moral clarity is the basis for countless decisions that are subject to human error, personality issues, patient compliance, reaction to illness, cultural differences, implicit trust, and random chance. For example, a bad clinical *outcome* despite a provider's best intentions falls into a gray area that we deal with all the time. For this reason, many health providers practice defensive medicine which substantially increases the cost of care.

Years ago, an oncologist addressed our group of interns and residents and explained that defensive medicine is understandable as a default, but we should not practice medicine in fear of making mistakes. "A good clinical decision," he said, "regardless of the outcome, can be justified and defended." He also assured us that a patient is less likely to sue a provider who fosters a relationship of trust and caring, even if something goes wrong. Conversely, a bad relationship between patient and provider is a powder-keg for lawsuits that ignite at the drop of a hat.

Our sage attending practiced 45 years with his share of adverse clinical outcomes, which is expected in the field of oncology, yet he was never served with a lawsuit. One could argue that he was just lucky or a great doctor, or perhaps he was right about the importance of relationships and trust.

"Confidence and hope do more good than physic"

-Galen

Claudius Galen, a Greek physician in the year 180 AD, asserted that a patient's trust in a caregiver is important as medicine itself. And it is no less true today. When a patient is assured that the care they are about to receive will be helpful, their *trust* in the physician goes a long way toward a successful outcome. It is evident in real time, as long as the treatment is good and the provider's words are true. How does this pertain to moral ambiguity? Let's take a look:

Medical decisions, like all other decisions, are subject to bias and error. This is the subject of fascinating work in heuristics that explain why people are wrong so often, even when they think they're right. In medicine, there are four principal reasons for mistakes:

Limited fund of knowledge (ignorance, or if the correct answers are simply unknown)

Incorrect information (poor source material, lab error)

Rush to conclusion (impulsive, too busy, deadlines)

Bias (gender, racial, socioeconomic)

A common situation in which caregivers are wrong when they *think* they're right is *overconfidence* despite a *limited fund of knowledge*. Also known as the "Dunning-Kruger effect," a caregiver may be unaware of his or her own limitations. This may be due to a relative lack of experience, poor study habits, arrogance, poor clinical acumen, or lack of accurate or available information. Any or all of these possibilities can lead to a medical error, yet there are caregivers who embody these common flaws and care for patients every day. It sounds scary but with proper safeguards in place it's not as bad as it seems.

Case in point: the phrase, "If you hear hoofbeats, think of horses not zebras" was coined in the 1940's by Dr. Theodore Woodward, a reminder that common things occur more commonly. *Experienced* doctors who practice with this in mind save time and money, and make the correct diagnosis more often, too. On the other hand, a new medical student who's just heard a lecture about malaria causing fever and an enlarged spleen is evaluating a patient in the clinic with presumed mononucleosis. Considering the clinical presentation and the student's limited fund of knowledge, he makes a tentative diagnosis of malaria.

In this example, the diagnosis of malaria was made because of inexperience, and our eager medical student would be wrong 99% of the time. But if the patient's recent trip to Africa was overlooked by everyone else and the red blood cell analysis showed parasites, our medical student would get a gold star for making a brilliant diagnosis. Sometimes the hoofbeats we hear come from a zebra. Far more commonly, correct answers are found by those who pay attention to details. Providers who take the time to listen, unrushed, with an open mind, are more likely to be correct.

"Nobody does wrong willingly"

-Socrates

When inexperienced caregivers are told they did something wrong, they may be surprised or embarrassed at first. From this we observe their character and willingness to learn, and in ourselves an opportunity to teach.

It is not an understatement to suggest that in medicine there is little room for mistakes, big or small; we all recognize the importance of good clinical outcomes, the high stakes involved (especially in critical care) and the medical-legal cloud that hovers over a poor outcome. This is why providers are insured to the gills for malpractice—because even defensible, unintentional errors can ruin a caregiver's career. How's that for pressure?

On any given day a Major League baseball player can be charged with an error and it's not even a speedbump in his career. That's nice for an athlete, but I've had friends in the field of medicine who'd checked every box of diligence, intelligence, and superb training, and they were still raked over the coals by an unforgiving legal system. Without exception, their mistakes were not out of negligence as much as being in the wrong place at the wrong time or with the wrong patient or just the wrong clinical outcome. How's that for moral ambiguity? In my own career I was never served with a malpractice suit, partly because I always worked with a quality team, but I'm sure it also boiled down to good luck. Unless, as our beloved oncology mentor had taught so well, a good doctor-patient relationship matters in ways beyond jurisprudence.

Like it or not, moral ambiguity includes every sphere of healthcare—whether you're an EMT, LPN, phlebotomist, pharmacist, dentist, or cardiologist—those who accept responsibility for the well-being of another will subject themselves to risk. It's part of the job. Unlike firefighters, healthcare workers don't run into burning buildings to save lives; instead, it's a slow burn that we endure for years, a frenetic pace with high acuity and uncertain outcomes. We do it regardless of a patient's financial status or political leanings or failure to pay child support, or if they cut you off during the drive into work this morning. Moral ambiguity means that providers with baggage care for patients with even more baggage. That's a lot to unpack, but the task is made easier when the priority is kindness.

In the criminal justice system, the cops get the bad guys and a prosecutor's job is to seek justice by exposing their behavior. But in healthcare it's the *opposite*. Providers are trained to recognize the moral failings of our patients and *set them aside*. We set aside their character flaws and *withhold judgment* in order to first *help* them. One can say that approach, itself, is morally questionable. I remember looking down at the swastika tattoo of a patient whose tennis elbow I was carefully injecting. It was not my place to do anything but provide quality care.

Disagreements abound in discussions of morality. In the right-to-life debate we recognize that some will defend a woman's right to choose and others will defend the life of the unborn—and the ironic thing is that both parties in this contentious debate see their own beliefs as unambiguous. In medicine we are trained to tolerate the opinions of patients and coworkers—not necessarily to *respect* the opinions with which we disagree, but to withhold judgment and keep them out of the conversation. There are enough subjects available to nurture a good relationship between patient and caregiver without bringing up the radioactive stuff.

Ultimately, *picking your battles* is a choice we make every day. It is part of being civil. Those who cannot accomplish this must ask themselves why it is necessary to be confrontational or why they must be right about everything? I remember laboring with this when I was much younger and I've since learned that people who need to be right about everything are insecure and not as smart as they think. I've also learned that a good listener who demonstrates kindness will engender more respect and accolades than being the smartest person in the room.

Dos and Don'ts:

If you are a patient with a medical appointment, remember the clerical staff that greets you has a job that is more difficult that it appears, including checking your insurance information, updating contact information, adhering to HIPPA requirements, tending to demands that have nothing to do with you, such as ringing phones, messages, and requests from other providers. So be nice and understanding and they will be nice to you.

Once you are checked in, a medical assistant or LPN will bring you into the exam room to check your vital signs, update medications and allergies, inquire about the reason for your visit and any other pertinent information. This is another opportunity for you to be nice, not only because it's the right thing to do, but because it will serve you well in the eyes of the clinical team. Please know that a medical staff notices the cranky, difficult patients, and they comment about other patients with phrases such as "Isn't she nice?" or "Isn't he a nice guy?" As much as it shouldn't matter in the grand scheme, these fleeting observations might influence a staff member when it's time to return a phone call or whether they go the extra mile to promptly contact a pharmacy or an insurance company on your behalf. It may sound unfair, but healthcare workers are prone to the same human flaws and lapses of favoritism as other well-meaning individuals.

On the provider side, there are many more dos and don'ts. Here's an example: say it's a busy Tuesday afternoon and you've already spent more time with Ms. Q than you'd expected. She had dozens of questions about her condition, needed extra reassurance about a relatively safe treatment, and now you're beginning to run behind. Your staff is getting restless and several patients are backed up, waiting to see you, so after a few encouraging, conclusive remarks, you inch toward the door and reach for the doorknob, but she does not say farewell; rather, she insists there are several more issues that she wishes to discuss with you.

Your response to Ms. Q will likely depend on the kind of day you're having. You might suggest to her that the remaining issues (whatever they may be) can be discussed during her next visit. You can explain that you've already spent time with her and other patients are waiting. Or you can do the right thing, which is to settle back into her private world where the two of you are the only ones who matter—because unless you do, she will not be happy—and if she leaves the office unhappy, then all the work you've done to gain her trust and confidence will be for naught.

Granted, there are times when you've had it, when you're certain that one less needy patient in the practice won't matter, but if you let her leave the office without addressing her concerns you will instantly regret it. Perhaps next time you won't pack your schedule so tightly that it creates undue tension. Here are a few other dos and don'ts:

Do: Keep in mind that patients may be anxious or afraid in the medical setting—consider this before you judge their attitude.

Answer all pertinent questions, explain lab results and relevant treatment options.

Help with peripheral issues (disability forms, Return-To-Work notes, FMLA forms, DMV forms, records release, etc.)

Respect privacy and HIPPA regulations—try to minimize traffic in the exam room (medical students, interns, scribe, excess family). Be extra careful with sensitive documents and phone messages.

Detect signs of abuse, depression, drugs – document and refer if necessary.

Casually inquire about family, lifestyle, hometown, or work-related issues—this helps to cultivate a bond and may help with clinical decisions, too.

Comfort and reassure—it's okay to offer a hug (or return a hug) if your patient is upset.

Go to a funeral—it's fitting to pay your respects to certain patients and their family members.

Don't: Make patients wait too long—nobody likes to wait more than half an hour in a waiting room. Get help or lighten the schedule if necessary.

Bring your personal anger or remnants of a bad day into the exam room

Take personal phone calls while in the exam room

Gossip or complain about your personal life, politics, religion, or salary—but allow your patient to privately discuss these issues if they wish.

Admonish a staff member in front of a patient

Disparage a colleague in front of a patient

Frighten a patient with hyperbole about how things can go terribly wrong—be kind and objective without adding undue anxiety.

Talk about your own sexual experiences, even if a patient asks.

Give or lend money to a patient.

Lie, if you're asked to fudge a document, jury duty request, insurance, disability or out of work form.

*

Clarity in a crazy world

Dealing with a minor inconvenience should be a manageable task for any mature adult with basic coping mechanisms—but when the hectic pace of a hospital ward gets maddening and nothing is going right, the limits of patience are tested. For a lucky few, the ability to handle stress is a default reaction that requires no special adjustment; for others the capacity to take a deep breath and carry on is done carefully. Of course, there are times when the challenge is simply overwhelming. Just ask the stressed parent of a toddler whose public tantrum is forcing dubious looks, or a new teacher on the first day of an unruly class in an overcrowded school, or a nursing student assigned to a busy surgical ward where patients are crashing and angry family members have a million questions. They all discover the truth that no job worth doing is easy.

In these situations, equanimity—remaining confident and composed—helps those who deal with frightened, confused, angry or aggressive individuals. After all, we have little influence over the behavior of others if we cannot first control our own, and one of the best ways to accomplish this is to become a skilled listener. By listening carefully, we can determine what others need or why they're upset. In healthcare, patients are often afraid; they may not understand what's wrong with their bodies or why they're there. Others may be angry about an issue that has little to do with their health, such as an administrative glitch or a misunderstanding that happened earlier, but if you listen, they will tell you what is wrong. By listening to them you are already earning your paycheck, and if finding the correct answer takes time, that's okay.

A good caregiver knows how to focus on patient care and leave the background noise aside. How does that happen? It's a matter of parsing the available choices that range from chaos to cure and knowing how to deal with each obstacle along the way. For example, why would I get frustrated by a sick patient or a crazy schedule when I already know that it's just part of the job? No matter who is crying or complaining, my job is the same. I am there to help.

"Kindness is more than deeds. It is an attitude, an expression, a look, a touch. It is anything that lifts another person."

-Plato

More about Clarity

Healthcare workers are constantly faced with differing opinions, yet we don't argue very much, at least not openly in front of patients. A public argument would be disruptive and counterproductive. What happens when we disagree? To begin, a worthwhile dispute involves at least two differing points of view that vary from workable to insurmountable. If there is no hope for a resolution, a stubborn impasse can escalate to a pointless argument. When this happens, nobody listens anyway.

Then there is clarity. A clear thinker can see *both sides* of an argument. When clarity of thought is present, one might be persuaded to shift from a given point of view to another. This happens when opinions and attitudes aren't static; that is, when points of view are open to flexibility and learning. When you consider that *opinions* reflect information, ideas, and experiences that are fluid and dynamic, subject to change based on events around us or by others whose opinions impress us most, it begins to make sense. It happens all the time in the field of medicine when we set our egos aside to find the best solution to a given problem.

When a patient is presented at a conference or during rounds or an impromptu curbside consultation, an exchange of ideas and opinions can lead to collective brainstorming and (sometimes, hopefully) a moment of inspiration to the benefit of all. This is where *learning* happens. Anyone who believes there is only one correct solution to a given problem is less likely to learn. Humility, curiosity, and clarity are the keys to learning new things.

"It is impossible for a person to begin to learn what he thinks he already knows."

-Epictetus

The Stoic words of Epictetus, a Greek philosopher who died 2,000 years ago, still resonate today. Kindness begins with humility, which includes the ability to keep an open mind about learning new things, welcoming others' opinions, and showing respect for ideas that may differ from yours. Kindness is an asset in the current climate of personal and political differences that have increasingly defined our social circles and attitudes. For this reason, at least within the healthcare arena, it helps to move beyond petty issues and focus on the greater task at hand.

This brings us back to the value of *equanimity.* The best caregivers are less likely to be blinded by emotion—not only wayward passions such as anger, jealousy or hate, but character-driven issues that inspire puerile pranks, romantic distractions, excess risk-taking and other irrational behaviors that affect clinical judgment. Clarity of thought leads to responsible decision-making and sets a good example for trainees. It is easier to reassure a patient and offer quality care when there isn't a whirlwind of excess emotion swirling about. It bears repeating: kindness does not require an effusive smile or overt gesticulations, just a sincere connection.

Active listening

I remember the comedian George Carlin once explained in an interview that he loved people as individuals but less so when they coalesced into groups. Fortunately, in the confines of an exam room, caregivers and patients are usually alone, together, with the presumption of privacy. It's a great way to get to know someone.

Yet for some reason, certain providers find it difficult to bond with their patients. I've been to countless medical meetings where well-attended plenary sessions addressed the theme "dealing with the difficult patient." The title always intrigued me because dealing with people should be a skill that is learned well before medical training. Out of curiosity I once poked my head inside a session and I was amazed by the number of physicians taking notes. Did they expect an algorithm? I could have told them the best way to deal with anyone is to *listen*.

Giving a patient (or anyone) your undivided attention should not be hard to do, yet for some it poses a challenge. During the course of a busy day, our thoughts drift, we get distracted, and the details are lost. On the contrary, staying focused, listening willfully, and avoiding miscues are all part of taking a successful patient history. With practice, the payoff for provider and patient is worthwhile. Whether you got up on the wrong side of the bed, or the car didn't start, or your sports team lost a nailbiter, you must listen attentively to the details of your patients' lives.

It bears reminding that healthcare workers have a unique opportunity (and responsibility) to listen to highly personal problems. This underscores the contract of trust that must be *earned*—not unlike the robes of a judge or the collar of a priest—because credibility is essential to the task of healing. It is a privilege that serves both providers and patients well. Patients willingly confer their trust to healthcare providers because they **want** to get better, and caregivers, in turn, work hard to earn their trust and share in a successful outcome.

To succeed in healthcare, both parties should share the goal of *listening* to one another. It's how barriers break down and communication happens. It requires an environment that is conducive to listening, preferably a private space with few distractions. Active listening is a give-and-take between speaker and listener in which verbal and non-verbal cues are used, and attentiveness is demonstrated with proper feedback. This closes the loop so that both parties know they have been heard and understood. It's a subtle dance.

Among the non-verbal clues in patient care are eye-contact, a smile (when suitable), attentive posture, a sympathetic nod, and a proper response to show that you're tuned in. It's okay if most of the listening is lopsided on the part of the provider—it may be less interactive but we *want* the patient to talk about themselves. A bond is forged by listening thoughtfully so the patient can feel heard. That's how healing begins. Providers who mostly preach are less effective.

"The reason we have two ears and one mouth is to listen more and talk less."

-Diogenes Laertius (230 AD)

Over the years, healthcare providers gather experience and confidence that allows them to offer reassurance when appropriate. They learn how to pick out the few patients each day who may be in trouble while reassuring the rest not to worry. When a patient hears the words "you'll be fine," their spirits brighten right away. In some cases, they begin to feel better, too. It may sound easy to reassure a patient, but it takes years of practice. The hard part is being correct; the easy part is being kind.

Patient Satisfaction

The essentials of patient satisfaction can be broken down as follows:

1) Good communication with providers and staff, responsiveness, availability, access to test results, reasonable wait times.

2) Clear instructions regarding treatment, risks/rewards, warning signs, how/when to follow up

3) Clean office/hospital environment, professionalism, safety

4) Kindness/attitude, language support, dealing with complaints

5) Answers to common questions, billing, pharmacy, referrals

6) Quality outcomes

The above guidelines may help garner patient satisfaction, although they are hardly comprehensive; the more crucial elements are written between the lines. Patient satisfaction is built on trust and rapport for which there is no simple algorithm.

The *National Institute for Health and Care Excellence* (NICE) provides guidelines for healthcare practitioners that include quality standards, patient experience, individualized care, and useful tips for patient satisfaction. Details are available online.

Managing Expectations

Patient satisfaction is key to optimizing medical care, provider reputation, and the business of medicine, and one of the best ways to achieve patient satisfaction and *avoid patient frustration* is to *manage expectations.*

Expectations govern our reactions to random events. If you bite into a sour pickle expecting a cucumber the taste might be repulsive—but if you had *expected* a sour pickle, the taste would be just right. In either case, it's the same pickle, only your expectations were different.

Similarly, our reactions to life's events are tailored by expectations. In healthcare, *expectations* are aligned with *prognosis,* and the many permutations of illness, treatment options, and results of decision-making affect each event that unfolds. Perhaps a bite into that sour pickle did not unnerve you because you were expecting it, but now at the front of the office, a belligerent patient is railing against your staff because of an ill-timed misunderstanding. You are fully aware that these things happen and it's nothing personal, yet how you maintain your composure will determine the outcome of this mess. Instead of seeking confrontation, you are prepared to offer assistance. That's just one example of a provider being prepared and managing the possibilities. In terms of patient satisfaction, the expectations are reversed.

Whether you work in a medical office or hospital ward, it helps to have *written policies* in place to govern patient expectations. For example, a patient who calls the office requesting a same-day appointment (which may not be feasible or necessary) needs to understand that only certain requests can be honored. Similarly, requests for pain medication by phone or an antibiotic called in to the pharmacy without being seen in the office can be problematic. By managing expectations, patients are less likely to become frustrated or feel that others are getting preferential treatment. Staff members should be ready to share guidelines that may include:

1) Requests for *same-day appointments* made after 10:00AM will be triaged depending on provider availability and the urgent nature of the problem.

2) Requests for *antibiotics* must be made *in-person.*

3) P*rescriptions for pain medication* must be given *in-person* if not seen in the office during the past 30 days.

These are just a few examples that help a busy office staff manage patient expectations *before* any sore feelings emerge. Likewise, it helps to clarify certain issues *before* a patient sees the provider, such as billing issues, co-pays, ABN's (advanced beneficiary notices), and alternative payment options, if necessary. Medical care is expensive and sore feelings regarding a misunderstanding of payment policy can be prevented. Furthermore, to limit excessive phone calls to the office, providers should answer all questions and take a moment to clarify specifics such as diagnosis, prognosis, monitoring requirements, and the need for follow up. Even better, a patient will benefit from being given hand-written instructions when possible. Most of all, providers and staff should earn trust, listen carefully, speak slowly, show respect, and never be dismissive.

The *results* of medical decisions include a fair number of possible outcomes—a *smaller number than one might think*—and this is where *pre-educating* a patient can make a big difference. For example, most complications and perceived setbacks are temporary speed bumps that require no treatment at all, whereas certain innocuous symptoms are actually warning signs of serious illness. This information should be shared. Once a diagnosis is made and treatment is rendered, anticipating the timing of recovery or the emergence of unwanted complications is essential for *patient communication,* so that patients know when it's necessary to call for help and when it's okay to wait. I picked a few examples in no particular order:

There was a time not long ago, say before 1990, when a woman with Lupus was strongly advised against becoming pregnant because it was felt to be too dangerous (for mother and baby). Consequently, a diagnosis of Lupus was devastating to a young woman whose heart was set on becoming a mother. Now, things are different. With greater awareness, a woman of child bearing potential is educated about the risks of pregnancy in Lupus, the precautions taken, the screening required including specific labs, fetal ultrasound, fetal non-stress testing, anticoagulation when appropriate, the continuation of medication such as hydroxychloroquine, and avoidance of certain medication such as mycophenolate to increase the odds of a healthy outcome.

Rarely there is a need for acute intervention, but what has changed more than anything is that the *expected outcome*, once ominous, has become more optimistic. That's good news for mother and baby. The risks are better known and monitored carefully, and a young couple can weigh and measure these risks with an open mind in order to make a careful decision. There are occasional tragic outcomes, but the same can be said in the absence of Lupus, too. There are occasional false alarms—variations in blood pressure, urine protein, hematocrit, deceleration of fetal heart rate—that may or may not pertain to Lupus at all, and these things keep everyone on their toes. The important thing is that all hands are on-deck until that baby is born, because having a healthy baby is the desired outcome, Lupus or not, and wisdom, experience, and kindness propel a caregiver's efforts at reassurance that anxious parents so desperately need.

A far less serious situation where expectations come into play is a simple but painful condition known as *gout*. Previously considered a plight of aristocrats, the tables have turned in America where low-income patients are more likely to be obese beer-drinking enthusiasts with diabetes, gout, and other metabolic issues.

Patients treated for gout are usually given anti-inflammatory medication, dietary advice, and a prescription for a uric acid lowering agent that reduces the risk of subsequent painful flares—*however the benefits are not always seen right away*. On occasion, gout patients stop taking their prescribed medication as soon as they feel fine, or the opposite—they flare early on and assume that the treatment will never work. For these reasons, patients with gout must be educated about the anticipated *course* of their condition so they will be more likely to comply with treatment and less likely to experience recurrent flares. A similar approach helps address problems such as smoking, drug use, excess alcohol, or eating too much of the wrong foods.

Expectations are about the future, and risk modification is about *behavior*, simple as that. With patience and kindness, healthcare providers who spend a little extra time explaining *choices and outcomes* can make a worthwhile difference.

Beer and baseball

Jamal was a skilled diesel mechanic whose main temptation was beer. He enjoyed three or four at night and a six-pack or more on Saturdays and Sundays. His uric acid level hovered around 7 if he took his medication, assuming he could limit the steak and shrimp in his diet. Whenever his favorite baseball team won, he celebrated with a few extra beers. When they lost, he drank even more, hence the *flares of gout* between April and October.

Jamal and I liked to talk about baseball, not just the standings or who won the night before, but things like OPS, WAR, bunting strategy, ghost-runner controversy, and the other armchair GM issues. He had a deep knowledge of the game and enjoyed bringing up the names of players long forgotten, if only to make a point.

Caring for Jamal's gout would have been a breeze were if not for his eating and drinking habits. I explained that he had to drink less beer, more water, reduce the meat and shellfish, and take his pills every day—simple things that could stop his gout attacks forever. But nothing is easy as it sounds. His baseball team struggled with injuries, fielding errors, mental miscues, overzealous umpires, and plain old bad luck, which translated into more 6-packs and more visits to my office. It would have been nice if his team had hired a new general manager or at least a few guys who could hit the ball. Since that wasn't happening, it was time for another talk.

Jamal was not afraid of getting gout attacks; they hurt like hell but he carried on and considered them temporary setbacks. As far as he was concerned, a gout attack was treatable with the right pills or a cortisone shot to the joint. The problem, as I had explained to him, was not one gout attack or two gout attacks, but the cumulative effect of multiple gout attacks resulting in destructive arthritis. Eventually he would have chronic pain in his feet, toes and ankles that could be permanent.

I told him it was a matter of preventive care—the same way we prevent heart attacks and strokes—that the gout attacks had to stop. Still, Jamal knew that gout was not life-threatening like a heart attack, and he did not appear concerned. The mischievous look in his eye was a signal to me that a cold beer was waiting in the fridge.

Rather than striking out again, I tried to persuade him by framing the problem in baseball terms. "You remember the pitcher David Wells? He had gout attacks pretty bad, even missed a few starts because of it."

"I don't root for the Yanks or the Blue Jays," he said.

"That's not it," I said. "The point I'm trying to make is that the pros practice good habits every day so they can be ready for anything.

That's what Wells had to do, and it's what I want you to do, reduce the red meat in your diet, lose 20 pounds, drink more water, and cut back on the beer." I looked directly into his eyes. "You're not that young anymore, Jamal. And it's not just about the gout, you're overweight too, at risk for heart attack, stroke and diabetes. My job is to keep you alive long enough to see your team win the World Series."

This time he perked up at the image. "Okay, you win. Tell me what I have to do."

*

New patients

"*Where did you grow up?*" is a question I ask sometimes during a new patient encounter. It allows me to learn about their background and it could serve as a launching pad to discuss other familiar things. In the confines of the exam room, patients like to talk about themselves—it's what they know best—and I get to divulge a little about myself too, if they ask. This sharing of information helps forge a useful bond without betraying any professionalism.

Later on, I might ask "*What do you do for fun?*" It's an easy way to explore a patient's personal interests if they are willing to go in that direction. It also helps me determine if they participate in sports or exercise or if they prefer more sedentary pursuits. More importantly, the question pulls them away from the formality of the exam table to a comfortable space with answers that range across a wide spectrum of possibilities: music, crafts, gardening, reading, spending time with family, or a multitude of lifestyle interests that open new doors to conversation. If you think this kind of information is irrelevant, I promise you it's not. Friendly, superficial talk is an opportunity for patient and provider to let their guards down and reveal themselves in ways that are spontaneous and therapeutic.

The essentials of medical data such as pulse, blood pressure, body weight, heart & lung sounds, etc. are obtained and recorded—drug allergies, medications, hematocrit, creatinine, EKG—that's the easy part. The real challenge is getting the *story*. A quality caregiver knows this, not because it's taught in medical school but because it's learned in real time. I like to record this information in the medical record for future use at the end of the HPI (history of present illness) so I can refer to it and bring it up casually during an opportune moment, sometimes a month or a year later: "How's your Golden Retriever?" or "Have you been to your grandson's Lacrosse games lately?" The instant reconnection nurtures the healing process and enhances the visit for both patient and provider. It's a great way to spend the day, to pass the time, and forge lasting relationships during the course of a career.

Curiosity

Curiosity is a gift that keeps caregivers involved and connected to patients; it drives empathy, humor, and pathos, all present at the core of the human condition. In particular, curiosity about the *feelings of others* provides an opportunity to stop thinking about ourselves for the moment; it's a fitting distraction against a cynical, nihilistic world. When the news of the day becomes too much to bear, caregivers can always count on others to *let them help*.

Those who *lack* curiosity find frustration in the helping professions, while those who *care* find satisfaction. In the world of healthcare, there are fulfilling roles for any and all who wish to participate—just ask a nurse's aide or hospice worker and they'll tell you about the lives they have touched.

Curiosity is the reason that good caregivers are good listeners. Tell me your problem and maybe I can help. How are you feeling today? I'd like to know. I'm interested.

"If your choices are beautiful, so too will you be."

-Epictetus

Self-esteem

At the low end of the confidence spectrum is *poor self-esteem*. Being under-confident is a dilemma for anyone who is still learning (which is all of us) and it is magnified in the health field where decisions are complex and many eyes are watching. The "Imposter Syndrome" is a phenomenon that primarily affects newcomers and perfectionists who feel anxious about serving in a high-functioning position, and despite having the intelligence and skill to be there, they may nonetheless believe their status is undeserved. It gets even worse when a sick patient dies. That's when young caregivers begin to question their own ability. How should they reconcile this?

The answer is *not* with feigned confidence—it's with humility and knowing when to get help—because patients will not accept a mistake made at their expense, nor do they want to hear a clumsy excuse about being new on the job; rather, they expect inexperienced caregivers to recognize their limits and wait for proper supervision.

Ultimately, learning to be a good caregiver takes years of experience built on character, repetition, success and *disappointment*. To a beginner this may sound daunting, but fortunately *the bar of expectation doesn't rise until it's supposed to.* When medical students follow me around and I toss a question in their direction, I don't expect them to know the correct answer (although I'm happy when they do). The questions serve as a launching pad, and the discussions that follow are for learning. In a few years they will ask the same questions to *their* medical students. It's a right-of-passage that has endured for centuries.

"Be tolerant of others and strict with yourself."

-Marcus Aurelius

Smart vs kind

Would you rather have a physician who is smart or kind? The answer is both, of course, but if you had to pick one attribute, which would it be?

The answer is *smart.* Clinical skills and intelligence are essential when choosing a healthcare provider, although surveys show that *kindness* consistently ranks high as well, even higher than the cost of care, travel distance, waiting times, and other factors.

In which type of medical practice does *kindness* matter most? The answer depends on whether you believe certain disciplines require more interpersonal connection for success. A pathologist, for example, can be kind as a kitten, but in order to make the best contribution to the team it is more important to be technically skilled. Likewise, a radiologist is trained to recognize complex pathology and find hidden problems via sophisticated technology. Kindness notwithstanding, it is crucial for such an expert to be skilled and accurate.

A surgeon's demeanor is important because patients count on them to be kind, confident and reassuring—some would even argue that a surgeon's kindness can promote a more favorable outcome (see below)—but the converse, a friendly surgeon lacking technical proficiency, can be problematic. Fair or not, patients tend to rate the kindness of their surgeon based on clinical *outcomes* as much as anything. For example, if a hip replacement turned out great, the orthopedic surgeon would get extra points for being nice, too. On the other hand, a poor surgical outcome or a postop complication, even if it wasn't the surgeon's fault, may be remembered as a personal grievance against the caregiver. Even the kindest surgeons have been dragged into court, their reputations sullied, or worse.

Certain practitioners are judged by kindness as much as intelligence. For example, primary care physicians, pediatricians, nurses, geriatricians, and others are often evaluated as such. I am not suggesting that their clinical competence is less important than other disciplines, but when office visits are non-urgent and routine in nature, the kindness of the caregiver is emphasized.

Another reason that kindness matters is the *therapeutic value of kindness itself.* This was described in an article in the NY Times (1/22/19) by Lauren Howe & Kari Leibowitz titled, "Can a Nice Doctor Make Treatments More Effective?" in which research in the psychiatry department at Stanford University demonstrated that having a provider who is warm and reassuring can actually improve your health. They pointed out that a physician's words are more powerful than most people realize. Not only the words, but the tone as well. For example, the phrase, "You'll be fine" if uttered in a terse, dismissive tone can nullify one's attempt at reassurance, whereas the same words spoken sincerely are more likely to be therapeutic. Put differently, when providers are competent but not warm (business-like, distant) the *perception* of their competence tends to diminish as well. This halo effect is common in medicine—nicer doctors are perceived to be more competent by patients and colleagues, and vice versa. Fair or not, that's just the way it is. The NY Times article suggests that the benefit of kindness isn't merely subjective; the *clinical outcomes are measurably better* as well. It shows us how important it is for providers to connect with patients, and that healthcare works best in an atmosphere of interpersonal connection.

I've observed brilliant colleagues who can recite the medical textbook inside and out, yet for some reason they scare the hell out of their patients by enumerating all the terrible things that can happen if a lab value is marginally outside the bell curve, if a patient doesn't comply with an innocuous medication, if a patient declines an obscure test, or merely asks for a second opinion. I promise you, 90% of patients will do fine (or not) regardless of whether their lab values are perfect or if they are 100% compliant with instructions. The reality is that a certain percentage will simply not take their prescribed medications properly. They will stop their antibiotic too soon, they will skip their evening dose of medication on occasion, and they might even miss a follow up office visit. How a physician deals with it makes all the difference in the world. Wagging a sanctimonious finger is not the answer. Thoughtful guidance is the way.

A quality caregiver diligently keeps track of essential details, monitors them carefully, picks out the patients who need prompt intervention, and reassures the rest. Along the way, it helps to be nice and considerate without unnecessarily frightening patients, rushing them, condescending, scolding, humoring, or patronizing them.

Let us also not overestimate the importance of every routine office visit. During the course of the day, a few red flags may be discovered and addressed, while the vast majority of health screenings serve to reassure patients and providers alike that all is well. What I'm trying to say here is that being kind should be easy for a provider to deliver while delivering quality care. It's about *caring while caring* for someone.

Back to the original question, is it more important for a healthcare provider to be smart or kind? Well, when you consider that during the course of a typical day 80% of medical issues are uncomplicated requiring little more than reassurance and monitoring, and the other 20% need some form of intervention, technical skill, or complex decision making, I would say (for the purpose of this book) that *both* kindness and intelligence matter a lot.

We all want a kind, competent professional at the helm. I wish I could tell you that 100% of providers fit the bill, but the actual percentage may disappoint you. Look at it this way, in an ideal world if 90% of healthcare providers are kind and 90% are smart (clinically astute and technically skilled), then the *odds of your provider being both kind and smart are roughly 81%.* That's 4 out of 5 doctors, and that's a generous assessment. The bottom line is this: If a patient is not satisfied with a doctor's demeanor *and* clinical skills, they have the option to move on—without a guarantee that they'll find someone better, at least not right away. Ultimately, there is no reason to settle for smart versus kind. There are many who can provide both.

Knowledge vs Experience

Which is more important, knowledge or experience? One could argue that experience is more important when engaged in an *activity* such as playing a sport or an instrument or performing a medical procedure. For example, you can know everything about the game of baseball, but unless you actually take the field and swing the bat, your knowledge can only go so far. Likewise, the first time you perform a medical procedure or run a code during a cardiac arrest can be shaky no matter how smart you are. There is no substitute for experience.

"Experience is the hardest kind of teacher. It gives you the test first and the lesson afterward."

-Oscar Wilde

Case in point: During medical school while studying for a pharmacology final, I felt pretty confident, so I urged a pharmacist buddy to ask me a pharmacology question. "Go ahead, ask me anything."

He tossed me a softball. "Okay, what is Lasix?"

And I was stunned.

Every practicing doctor knows that Lasix is the brand name for generic furosemide. But I wasn't a doctor yet, just a cocky, inexperienced medical student. It was my Ralph Kramden moment. I knew all about loop diuretics, how to use them and how they worked, but I lacked the real-world experience to know the brand names of generic drugs. I realized then, and appreciate now, that experience matters, and so does humility.

I would also argue that apprenticeships are lacking in society; whether you are a doctor, a mechanic, or a baker, your best bet is to set the text aside when the opportunity arises, find a mentor and tag along. If you happen to be a mentor in the medical field or elsewhere, be patient and kind to your students as you would hope for yourself.

"If they've made a mistake, correct them gently and show them where they went wrong. If you cannot do that, then the blame lies with you—or no one."

-Marcus Aurelius

Interpersonal Skills

One can tell by reading a medical progress note if a provider is connecting with empathy and concern, or if the note is merely an amalgam of data. Too often, I've observed the notes of medical students and young doctors that are little more than an impersonal checklist of factoids. For example, the *history of present illness* may look like this: Patient had a headache. Patient took an aspirin. Patient denied nausea. Patient went to urgent care. Patient this and patient that, and so on... This approach to the medical record delivers the essential points of data, but the style is numbing to the senses and fails to capture any feeling. That's not to suggest that the author of each medical note must be a Hemmingway or Faulkner, but the occasional use of a pronoun or a bit of nuance can help paint a better picture. I mean, we're talking about a person, not a broken refrigerator.

Granted, there are cultural aspects of this type of documentation, which is a different problem that is easily fixed. What I mean is it's okay to refer to *the patient* every now and then, but it's also helpful to remind the reader that the patient is a person whose life has changed measurably enough to seek medical attention. For example, the migraine headache in question interrupted something important, and this additional information clarifies and embellishes the complaint— she had to stop breastfeeding because the baby's crying was "*so painful she thought her left eyeball was going to explode.*" This type of description not only allows the reader to feel invested in the headache, but in the life of *the person* with the headache. It's a humanist style that works well in the medical record.

Students and interns who follow me in the office and on hospital rounds witness this type of approach to note-writing that includes a measure of humanity, even when discussing such routine presentations as diabetes, high blood pressure, back pain, etc. The selective use of pronouns such as he or she (or they) illuminate the note better than "patient this" and "patient that." A written portrayal of *how* the presenting complaint affects someone's life adds color to the description, and the added backstory helps the provider (or anyone else reading the note) get up to speed for the next visit. These details may not seem important to a busy caregiver, but trust me, it means a lot to those who depend on us. Their stories are significant, and we can provide context on their behalf in the medical record.

Reassurance

During the course of a busy day, the art of comforting a *frightened* patient is not the same as tending to a *needy* patient. Every medical office has a roster of patients who push the limits of tolerance by calling too frequently with minor concerns just to be reassured. That's not to dismiss their concerns—the concerns are real, at least to them—they fear a recurrence of minor shoulder discomfort or fleeting heartburn after a large meal requires another phone call to a medical office or a trip to an urgent care facility.

The problem is, whether they realize it or not, too many non-urgent phone calls are counterproductive to their own care, and even with proper triage and the best of intentions among caregivers it is difficult to see everyone who calls. Of course, each medical complaint must be taken seriously—one can never know when a twinge of heartburn is actually the onset of a heart attack—so the onus must be reasonably shared. If a patient decides that a complaint is severe enough to pick up the phone for help, the provider should be available to intervene or at least provide reassurance.

"Many are harmed by fear itself, and many have come to their fate while dreading fate."

-Seneca

Providers and staff should have an ample supply of patience for those who need frequent medical attention, but there are reasonable limits to the demands of the day. Sometimes the burden of anxiety, fear, somatization, drug-seeking, rudeness, bossiness, or simple neediness, can overwhelm a medical practice. Such patients may be unaware that they have become a source of frustration. In the setting of private health insurance, Veterans Affairs, Medicare and Medicaid, it rarely costs the patient much (or nothing at all) to call with questions and concerns.

It begs the question, what is a provider's obligation to answer each question? Is there a limit to the number of calls per patient? Is there an appropriate amount of time before a provider must respond? How and when is triage performed, and by whom? If a patient calls with a headache, is there an algorithm to determine if it's a migraine, a brain tumor, or a hemorrhage? In the harsh reality of the current medical-legal world, these questions are asked all the time.

Put simply, most medical practices divert all true emergency phone calls to 911 or the nearest Emergency Department or urgent care facility by saying so right away at the recorded telephone greeting.

With that disclaimer, a patient may ultimately reach a clerical person or leave a message to state their question or concern. Assuming that voicemails are taken at least hourly, the medical clerk notifies the Medical Assistant or nurse, who considers the acuity of the problem and brings it to the attention of a provider for a response. The point is to answer the multitude of medical questions that arrive throughout the day, refill prescriptions, calm an anxious patient in a reasonably expedient manner, and to act quickly for all matters that require prompt attention. The best providers treat all patients with the same compassion they would provide for a family member—and it is remarkable how the frustrations of the day tend to dissolve when kindness is applied to helping people and handling their concerns.

And there is no expiration date—patients remember acts of kindness months and even years later. They're happy to remind us about things we might have said or done (even if we cannot remember). It's remarkable how caregivers affect patients that way. A single act of kindness can have a lasting effect.

Our visit to the eye doctor

Not long ago, my wife awakened with an unexplained worsening of the vision in her right eye. It was a Friday morning around 7:30AM and she'd already made an appointment to see the eye doctor the following Monday. But she looked afraid and unsure if it was okay to wait another three days until her scheduled appointment.

There were red squiggly lines in her right visual field that were punctuated by bright flashes of tiny lightning bolts, more than the usual floaters she had previously experienced, and it was getting worse.

As a devoted husband, my default position on such matters was to protect her and reassure her. But as a physician, I was out of my lane;

this was something for an expert to sort out. I was aware that a lot could happen in a short period of time: detached retina, stroke, optic neuritis, acute glaucoma, retinal vein thrombosis, or the most likely possibility that it was just a passing thing. It was too early in the morning to expect an answer at the doctor's office and I didn't want to spend the day in an emergency room, so I suggested that we wait another half hour for the office to open, then call to see if her doctor could see her today. Perhaps there was an opening or a cancellation.

I was tempted to make the call on her behalf and maybe drop my name as a local physician, but I thought better of it. Doing so might get her an appointment faster but the weird thing is that physician's spouses are sometimes treated excessively with more cautionary tests that lead to more tests and treatment, and that's the last thing we wanted. I sat by her side as she called and I could hear her conversation with the receptionist who explained that her doctor was in surgery all morning and did not have office hours on Friday afternoons. But instead of dismissing the request she said, "Let me get a nurse to ask you a few questions."

My wife described her symptoms to the nurse, the flashing lights and red squiggles in her right eye, and she was briefly put on hold. A moment later she was told that another ophthalmologist, Dr. Scartozzi, would see her this morning and could she come in right now?

Yes of course. We drove to the office building which was only fifteen minutes away. Upon checking in we were informed that there would be a bit of a wait since my wife was squeezed into the schedule. No problem, completely understandable. Over the course of the next 45 minutes, before seeing the doctor, she was escorted through a series of tests by two medical assistants including visual acuity, ocular pressure, and digital retinal photographs. At each step, the pertinent information was typed into her electronic health record. We were then guided to a new waiting area.

Fifteen minutes later a young doctor introduced himself and brought us into a room that was dimly lit with comfy chairs and elaborate equipment. I sat quietly as he reviewed the test results and meticulously examined my wife's eyes. The framed photos on his desk showed a young family. Several impressive diplomas on the wall did not go unnoticed.

At last, he sat back and said the retina looked fine and everything looked good, probably just floaters which should resolve over the next few weeks. He handed my wife a brochure on the subject and reviewed the warning signs that would require a prompt phone call at the earliest sign. He also explained what the vitreous is and what floaters are. He wasn't smiley or chatty, just kind, confident and professional. There was nothing phony about this young man who was at once busy and efficient. It was just what the doctor ordered, exactly what I had hoped for. We wished each other a nice weekend and stepped toward the checkout area to surrender a $35 co-pay. I checked my watch and saw it was 11:00AM.

Just a few hours earlier my wife had a disturbing change of vision in her right eye, and now she was walking beside me to the parking lot wearing sunglasses, calmly reassured, talking about what we should have for lunch. I thought about how fortunate we are, not only to be seen in such a timely fashion but to receive good news as well. Were we just lucky? Was it random happenstance that a specialist was available that morning?

I'd like to think our experience at the ophthalmologist's office was not only the model of expert care but an example of how calm efficiency and professional kindness can make a huge difference.

*

Three things

Each visit to a medical office includes one or more of the following: a routine health screening, an urgent complaint, an abnormal test result, a treatment regimen, monitoring a chronic condition, or maintaining wellness. In each situation, what is the obligation of a healthcare provider? The answer is basically two things—and I added a third:

1) make a correct diagnosis, if necessary

2) render proper treatment, if necessary

3) provide reassurance and advice

Accomplishing all three things becomes easier when basic kindness is included. To the jaded providers who are rolling their eyes, take a coffee break or a vacation and try to remember why you entered the field of medicine in the first place. If you've forgotten, or if your calling to medicine has changed from its original intention, remember that kindness and compassion are the driving forces behind everything good in healthcare.

The extra mile

It usually happens on Friday afternoon: a patient calls the office saying there isn't enough medication to last until Monday and insists that a prescription must be filled right away (despite our policy to allow 48 hours for such things). Of course, we do our best to get all pharmacy requests tucked in before the weekend because we don't want our patients to get upset, and we don't want the weekend answering service or covering physician to get additional calls, especially for narcotics or other scheduled drugs. So, what do we do? We address each request carefully and err on the side of compassion.

We do not want to deprive a patient in need any more than we want to be taken advantage of.

Additional sources of frustration are the late arrivals, late cancellations, and no-shows. In fairness, external circumstances are understandable—unexpected traffic, accident on the road, sick family member—and we do our best to fit everyone in. It's all part of keeping the customers satisfied. But there are times when a bunch of patients arrives too early or too late and the clerical staff is tested, especially if there's a limited crew due to a holiday or maternity leave or any number of events. It's a harsh reality for any service-related business from restaurants to department stores, that the creation of happy customers begins with service, a willingness to make adjustments and sacrifices during crunch time.

And then, ten minutes before the week is about to end, when the staff is tucking in loose ends and making giddy references to *happy hour*, an urgent add-on patient limps into the waiting area with a low-grade fever and a warm, swollen knee.

Everyone knows it could be serious, maybe a staph infection or acute gout. Maybe it's Lyme disease or a flare of rheumatoid arthritis. The only way to find out is to insert a sterile needle, remove a sample of joint fluid, analyze it under a polarizing microscope, check for crystals and bacteria, begin a culture in the lab, check for Lyme, uric acid, and other blood tests, and make a decision about treatment that may include an antibiotic, anti-inflammatory, or hospitalization.

All at once, the lighthearted atmosphere of the office is replaced by a desire to help this patient. Phone calls are made to alert the runners to the lab and the triage nurse at the ED. It remains unspoken that such urgencies occur in bunches. The notion of happy hour disappears. Drinks and laughter will not happen today, at least not right away. Hopefully no further surprises are looming on the horizon, like another hospital consult or more. During such times, the staff benefits from a level-headed office manager, an experienced nursing staff and a calm, confident provider. With everyone in place contributing, a good outcome is far more likely.

A professional staff should be ready with a good attitude, but there are limits and reasonable expectations. For example, the risk of too much extra work goes without saying, and a gradual decline in job satisfaction can lead to indifference, despair, or poor-quality care. Among the many causes in healthcare are overwork, mistreatment by a supervisor, personal problems, and much more. Overwork or mental fatigue due to excessive hours or complexity and acuity of patient care is a substrate for job burnout that creates an environment of frustration, mistakes, and unhappiness.

The best solution, like anything else, is prevention, but it's not always easy. It takes a perceptive supervisor to recognize the early trappings of frustration to make sure the demands of work are acceptable and vacations and personal time are carved into the schedules of all essential personnel.

At the peak of the COVID-19 pandemic, overwork and burnout were common and a shortage of caregivers was available to take the place of the fallen. This was a major dilemma for small towns with scant crews already overwhelmed by the demands of hospitalized patients, PPE (personal protective equipment) doffing and donning, long hours, insufficient resources, and constant personal risk. Many were heroic in their efforts, some died, others pressed on until they could bear no more, and the rest remained ineffectually bewildered.

Prior to the pandemic, healthcare workers were already subject to the risk of burnout, but COVID made it substantially worse. If anything, we must learn from the experience, avoid mistakes that were made, recognize the achievements of researchers who crafted effective vaccines in such a timely fashion, those in the public sphere who promptly rolled up their sleeves to get vaccinated, essential workers who kept society moving, and all frontline healthcare workers who showed up to help the sick and dying in such a selfless manner.

Essential workers

The field of medicine places caregivers at the center of people's lives, not merely as bystanders but *participants*. During the COVID-19 outbreak, doctors, nurses, EMTs, ambulance drivers, pharmacists, and hospital employees were among the first essential workers called to service.

Essential in this context means necessary and available: teachers, food workers, military service, delivery, construction, and other front-line workers were deemed essential during the pandemic as well. It was a difficult time for all, though it should be noted that healthcare workers—pandemic or not—are never *not* essential.

Dealing with Stress

Emotional stress and PTSD are responsible for more doctor visits than one can imagine. Among the clinical consequences of chronic stress are insomnia, fatigue, obesity, body pain, cardiac symptoms, irritable bowel, tension headaches and more. The psychosocial manifestations include anxiety, depression, spousal abuse, drug use, suicide, job loss and despair. A typical medical approach—blood tests, X-rays, prescription drugs, and so on—misses the boat by a mile. There is no shortcut to fixing the medical fallout of stress, no convenient pill to make everyone's troubles disappear.

Ultimately, the best treatment for stress (like most things in medicine) is *prevention*. Beyond that, optimal sleep, light exercise, and an anti-inflammatory diet are all helpful. Anxiolytics, cannabinoids, and SSRI medication are useful in selected cases. The problem is, by the time a stressed patient reports to a medical facility with somatic complaints, the symptoms are already entrenched and difficult to shut off. Successful treatment requires an approach that is rarely found in standard medical textbooks, partly because there is no simple algorithm, and it includes active listening, kindness, and patience. A few minutes of thoughtful inquiry can be helpful if the right questions are asked and the *stressed* patient is given a chance to talk.

The abundant sources of stress in society include every intractable demand and expectation placed on us (by ourselves and others), the cumulative angst over the past and future, the many external stressors thrust upon us, the unrealistic targets of success forged in our minds, plus global war, starvation, danger, illness, and so many more. Chronic stress abounds in every culture, triggered by all of the above, and no one is immune.

The epigenetics of chronic stress are fascinating and involve alterations of DNA expression that occur in response to external stressors such as danger, infection, poverty, pollution, injury and emotional abuse. This phenomenon dates back to the very first threats encountered by prehistoric man (dangerous elements, wild animals, starvation) up to the stressors of modern life (financial concerns, health issues, relationships, job-related stress, violence, and more). Then and now, unwanted stress triggers a secondary response in the immune system that fires up a host of inflammatory cytokines and invites chronic illness. Stress can bring an otherwise healthy person into the medical arena with chest pain, indigestion, headache, palpitations, or skin rash.

A condition known as Takotsubo cardiomyopathy or "broken heart syndrome" causes the heart muscle to abruptly weaken in response to sudden overwhelming stress, such as the unexpected loss of a loved one. This produces chest pain that resembles a heart attack or clinical features of congestive heart failure. It's a remarkable display of psychosomatic illness. In my practice, patients with inflammatory autoimmune conditions such as systemic lupus, psoriasis, Crohn's disease and MS are aware that stress may trigger a flare. The same thing can happen in those with Fibromyalgia, migraine headache, irritable bowel or chronic back pain. That's not to say that stress **causes** any of these conditions—but stress cuts into restorative sleep, activates inflammatory cytokines, and opens the door to episodes that may not have otherwise occurred.

When it comes to addressing the emotional needs of patients, medical providers themselves may be stressed, overbooked or nearly burnt out, so we must readily identify the red flags and help ourselves whenever possible. A successful approach to caring for people whose symptoms are driven by stress is not fully explained in standard medical textbooks, nor is it always learned in the classroom. So, what is a caregiver to do? Listening without judgment is a good place to start. From there, empathy and compassion set the tone. A few minutes of thoughtful inquiry can be invaluable if the right questions are asked and the patient is given a chance to talk. After that, it's just a matter of being a good human being. Many young providers are surprised by how therapeutic it can be to lend a compassionate ear, and how gratifying it is to simply be there for someone in need.

"When you are distressed by an external thing, it's not the thing itself that troubles you, only your judgment of it. And you can wipe this out at a moment's notice."

-Marcus Aurelius

More about Post-Traumatic Stress

If emotional trauma can produce unwanted physical and mental health symptoms, what about the *opposite*? Can kindness and comfort possibly address or even reverse the manifestations of PTSD? And if so, how and when does healing begin, and how long does it take?

So many times, I've pondered these questions. Not a day has ended without hearing at least one tragic account from a mistreated patient whose life was made unbearable by the cruelty of an event or the vile behavior of a family member, a coworker or a stranger. Verbal abuse, violence, rape, humiliation, crimes, accidents, war, hunger, and other random incidents can produce lifelong stress or post-traumatic stress—a hard-wired imprint on the brain—a loop of rehearsed memory that destroys the nascent sense of security we take for granted. The earlier the trauma (infancy, childhood) the deeper the wound, and the greater the damage the more difficult it is to repair.

But it's never too late to get help. What are some of the health issues that emerge in the aftermath of emotional trauma or chronic stress? They are numerous and highly individualized depending on the severity of the incident and the unique predisposition of each patient, such as genetics, conditioned tolerance, and support. This explains why there is no simple algorithm to dealing with the symptoms of PTSD. The circumstances and symptoms are rarely shared by any two patients. But we can categorize the clinical fallout of trauma to understand it better and perhaps begin to help patients recover one at a time. The common manifestations of chronic stress and PTSD include depression, anxiety, insomnia, eating disorders, drug use, unemployment, anger, hostility, cognitive issues, and more. Physical (somatic) complaints emerge from a phenomenon called central sensitivity, which amplifies the messages of neurotransmitters and creates a complicated symptom-complex that turns a person into a patient. Such maladies include fatigue, malaise, irritable bowel, headache, fibromyalgia, pelvic pain, dry eyes, atypical chest pain, chronic low back pain, and more.

The first mission of a caregiver is to exclude the common medical causes of a physical complaint, keeping in mind that it's possible to have more than one problem at a time. For example, a chronic whiplash injury can be exacerbated by an emotional trigger. It takes a kind ear and a lot of patience to sort through the details. A successful outcome begins with an attentive, active listener. In the course of a busy day, this is no small task. For this reason, it's important for both patient and caregiver to recognize the limitations of a single visit. In our impatient, prescription-oriented society, it helps to have a realistic timeline of recovery, and a provider must use multiple resources, if necessary.

"Any person capable of angering you becomes your master."

-Epictetus

Mental healthcare requires compassion.

There is growing concern that our modern rushed computerized medical environment has been destructive to quality mental healthcare. In fact, any barrier to forming a solid connection between patient and caregiver can interfere with a good clinical outcome. I would also argue that kindness helps, but it is not enough to foster a supportive mental health environment; in the sphere of behavioral medicine, *compassion* is key. Recall that, unlike kindness, which is measured by one's behavior, compassion is a built-in awareness of the distress of others, and a desire to alleviate their pain.

Freud referred to "the psychopathology of everyday life" as if to say that none of us is immune. Unfortunately, too many people think they are immune, believing instead, "that could never happen to me." This is where kindness and compassion go hand in hand—to see ourselves in each suffering patient—to offer relief beginning with a kind word.

As such, a mental health professional's connection with a struggling patient requires a foundation of non-judgmental advocacy; not merely with acts of kindness that can be routinely doled out, but a genuine desire to connect. If this raises the bar of expectations for mental health workers, that's perfectly fine, since the yearning to help is the same driving force that drew them to the field in the first place.

In deference to the advances in pharmaceuticals, there is still no substitute for one-on-one counseling by a compassionate therapist. I've worked closely with practitioners in the field of mental health to support the needs of patients with comorbid anxiety, depression, PTSD, bipolar disease, and schizophrenia, and it's becoming clear that the stigma associated with getting help for these conditions has lessened over the years. This may be due to quick access to information via social media and search engines, visible efforts by celebrities (Michael Phelps, Prince Harry, Glenn Close, Demi Lovato, and others), and a supportive young generation whose lives are more open and less secretive than those of prior generations. For these reasons and more, there is newfound hope for those with mental health issues, and many opportunities available to those who are ready to serve.

Treating chronic pain—an exercise in empathy

Fibromyalgia is a syndrome of widespread chronic pain and fatigue that affects millions of people during the prime of their lives. The common physiologic overlays of irritable bowel and migraine headache suggest an abnormal *central sensitivity of pain processing.* The syndrome can emerge after a triggering insult to the brain (physical, emotional, infectious, or environmental) in the setting of genetic predisposition with common psychosocial underpinnings such as anxiety, depression or post-traumatic stress. Any or all of these factors will affect restorative sleep, although the majority of fibromyalgia patients lack a specific psychiatric diagnosis. The insomnia that results can further amplify the symptom complex, particularly during periods of stress.

It appears that fibromyalgia lacks a single origin or unifying solution, which is why providers who care for patients with fibromyalgia must be particularly patient and considerate. Many questions arise during the course of treatment, underscoring the need to listen carefully and provide reassurance whenever possible. Providers and staff who keep an open line of communication with their patients get better results.

Fibromyalgia is invisible to all but those who care. Too often I've heard the diagnosis of fibromyalgia dismissed by skeptical colleagues who refuse to accept a diagnosis that is too difficult to define or measure, yet it's among the most common things we see.

For this reason, treating fibromyalgia requires empathy, patience, good communication skills, clinical insight, and kindness. Integrative care (combining the best of holistic and allopathic medicine) is the preferred approach to treating fibromyalgia addressing restorative sleep, chronic pain and mood issues, avoiding the use of narcotic analgesics, steroids or untested remedies, and to *first do no harm*. The pathophysiology and details of diagnosis and treatment are beyond the scope of this book. Years earlier when I published a book titled *Healing Fibromyalgia*, a deluge of patients came to see me for care. Having learned to care for patients with inflammatory autoimmune disease, I did not expect to see so many patients with chronic widespread pain in my general rheumatology practice, but looking back now I can say that it was a learning experience. It opened my eyes to the tremendous need for more answers and better treatment in this area.

A dear patient of mine with severe Fibromyalgia is a delightful woman named Linda. After witnessing the murder of a family member, her life changed immeasurably. First came bouts of anxiety and insomnia, followed by generalized body aches, digestive problems, lower back pain, depression and weight gain. From a healthy woman in her late twenties, Linda had become a poorly functioning thirty-two-year-old.

Linda's story has a happy ending, although it's important to point out that the improvement she experienced did not occur by treating each physical symptom. Instead, she took a step back to address her unresolved emotional trauma. Healing of this type can take years and requires the expertise of a mental health professional with a vested interest in this type of problem. A great book titled, "Healing Invisible Wounds" by Richard Mollica, MD provides a review of the subject and a path to recovery with stirring accounts of patients who'd survived unimaginable emotional trauma, including wartime violence, rape, torture, and humiliation.

Since I am neither a psychiatrist nor social worker, my role in helping Linda was to monitor her labs and medical issues, authorize a card for the use of *medical marijuana* (for symptoms of PTSD, insomnia, chronic pain, and digestive issues), correspond with her other specialists, encourage proper diet and aerobic activity, and most importantly to provide compassion during her recovery. For years I was an advocate for Linda's disability status and served as a resource for her many questions providing genuine concern, active listening, and supportive eye contact. I realize that one does not need an MD to do each of these things, which is proof that we all have the ability to help in some way.

Kindness is courage

A common misperception that kind people are timid or meek may appear true on the surface, but is quite the opposite in healthcare. Kindness in healthcare involves a willingness to take on the risks of exposure to illness, tend to urgent situations, and most of all assume *responsibility*. Acts of kindness require bravery by caregivers in underserved areas by social workers, pediatricians, EMT's, ambulance drivers, office managers, Emergency Department staffs, and more. Our friends at *Doctors-Without-Borders* can teach us a thing or two about bravery in the face of extreme poverty and war-torn landscapes.

What I'm trying to say is, in a society that glorifies gunslingers who blow people apart, the real heroes are those who put people back together—the orthopedists, trauma surgeons, physical therapists, counselors, and so on. Tireless obstetricians and midwives who take on unspeakable responsibility during the most tenuous moments of our lives deserve recognition for their efforts and availability 24/7. The social worker who enters a dangerous SRO building to assess the healthcare needs of a troubled client is daring beyond words. The pediatrician who stares down an abusive parent isn't just kind but unmistakably brave, too. If there's anything the COVID-19 pandemic revealed it's the sacrifices made by healthcare workers across the board, not only on the front lines, the ED, ICU, and medical wards, but the clerical staffers, cafeteria workers, janitorial staff, and other essential workers who knowingly exposed themselves to the risks of sickness and death. It never hurts to take a moment to recognize the boundaries of kindness that extend beyond comfort and care to include courage and a willingness to serve.

Early on during the COVID-19 pandemic we saw footage of healthcare workers in ICU and urgent care settings, and it was clear that the demands of the job were depleting the gusto from the most devoted employees. At the end of a grueling shift or months of serious decision-making, after witnessing one personal tragedy after another, it seemed the pandemic had taken its toll not only on the patients but the caregivers as well. Yet somehow, they endured for the greater good.

"Dig deep within yourself, for there is a fountain of goodness ready to flow if you keep digging."

-Marcus Aurelius

COVID-19 Nurses

At the peak of the COVID-19 pandemic, the role of *hospital nurse* had mutated into a nearly unrecognizable mission. What was already a difficult job had become an exercise of military-like acuity. Despite staff shortages, concurrent illness, and the ongoing risk of exposure, these essential workers remained financially undervalued. In my state of Connecticut, hospitals scrambling for nurses offered additional signing bonuses of $1,000, which was paltry compared to the incentives given to those in the financial and corporate worlds where one could work from home, out of harm's way.

Hospital nurses with expertise in infection control and critical care were irreplaceable during the pandemic, and they were ready to serve when legions of patients arrived frightened and short of breath. Most hospitals like ours split the clinical services geographically into COVID and non-COVID wards for optimal protection and efficiency. The brave nurses who tended to the sickest COVID patients early on (before vaccines) went above and beyond the call of duty. Day after day, doffing and donning PPE (personal protective equipment) left onlookers in awe. The indelible images of spectators applauding nurses and other hospital staff at the end of their shifts marked but a fraction of the appreciation felt by communities everywhere.

In our own medical office, nurses and medical assistants similarly endured everything asked of them. They wore N-95 masks and face shields all day, performed incessant hand-washing, changed gloves and applied sanitizer gel, asked crucial screening questions, provided answers, enforced policy, orchestrated remote/virtual visits, recorded vitals, and were repeatedly exposed to sick patients—all duties *added* to their pre-pandemic responsibilities. If a nurse or MA was infected with COVID-19, our office manager Vanessa Alves promptly found a replacement. Our tireless front-office staff, Connie Reinders, Isabel Ramos-DeSousa, Linda Wheeler, Joan Fiore, and Dillan Suggs carried on despite the added risks. And lest we forget, while the COVID-19 pandemic scorched the medical landscape, all other problems unrelated to COVID—stroke, heart disease, diabetes, cancer, and rheumatic disease—required treatment, too.

For a while it was a challenge to keep it together, yet there wasn't the slightest hint of discouragement. Our nurses and MAs confidently reassured patients, completed every required task, and returned home to their families at the end of the day. This went on for years without a lapse in attitude. If there was any sign of frustration or fatigue, they did not reveal it to the patients. Among these superb caregivers were Jennifer Heckmann, Jessica Edwards Palmieri, Tiffany Brett, Samantha Lopez, Chelsea LaBow Murphy, Essie Daniels, Crystal Jaquez and others who will forever have my gratitude.

*

Good mourning

Healthcare professionals are regularly called upon to help patients and families mourn the loss of a loved one. It is an unhappy task that never quite feels normal, yet somehow caregivers learn from each experience and are skilled at providing comfort.

One might ask, what is a reasonable amount of time to mourn? Six months? A year? Some people cry at the mere mention of the departed more than a year beyond the *typical* mourning period. But when is it too long? Surely, the loss of a young child can produce a source of melancholy that lasts forever. But if the death of a 94-year-old grandparent remains a source of despair and spontaneous tears a year later, I might be concerned—and if I observe this kind of despondence with clinical curiosity, what does it say about me? If I cannot feel genuine sympathy for each situation, am I being unkind? The answer is yes. So, rather than dwell upon the psychological underpinnings, I will do my best to understand and offer a compassionate ear. Tell me about your loved one. What was she like? How did she die?

From a medical standpoint, the physical manifestations of bereavement are common: altered appetite, reduced energy, interrupted sleep, body aches, or sometimes a flare of chronic illness. To offset these symptoms, a caregiver should watch for signs of depression or adjustment disorder, provide support by listening, encourage proper nourishment, sleep, exercise, hygiene, and social activity.

Upon seeing our share of death and grief, I wonder sometimes if doctors and hospital nurses (or soldiers, clergy, funeral directors, etc.) respond differently to such a thing. For better or worse, veteran caregivers know that death is a natural certainty, but we should be careful not to offer any frank pragmatism when a patient's loved one dies. There are many different ways to mourn, and each is an opportunity to offer comfort.

By the way, condolences also apply to a beloved pet. We may not feel the same immediate sense of loss when a tearful patient insists that her departed cat can never be replaced, but we should be able to allow her expression of grief. It's not only a nice thing to do, but it's the right thing to offer consolation, ask a question about the dear departed, offer a hug if that's what you feel they need, and spend an extra minute or two until they're ready. You'll be glad you did.

"It doesn't matter how good a life you've led, there will still be people standing around the bed who will welcome the sad event. But don't leave angry with them. Be true to who you are: caring, sympathetic, and kind."

-Marcus Aurelius

Practice makes perfect

The practice of medicine never ends, even when you think you're getting pretty good at it. Long after a medical or nursing degree is conferred, a daily rehearsal continues indefinitely toward the goal of mastery. And, like the practice of medicine, kindness must be practiced—by some more than others, of course—which means that caregivers must continually remind themselves (and each other) to be careful with their words and behavior.

When the chips are down and your mood is in the dumps, it helps to remember that your patients depend on you, and it's okay because you are practiced in the art. It means setting aside your personal distractions for the time being. A rookie caregiver may gripe to a patient that they're exhausted or upset about something, but a seasoned professional will offer kindness and support no matter what.

*

Selina

Lupus is an inflammatory autoimmune condition that affects women more than men, usually in the prime of their lives. Their stories are similar, yet no two are alike. What makes lupus particularly unsettling is its potential to be serious when everything seems to be going fine. Its onset can be vague with a mixture of fatigue, aching, rash, or kidney issues that remain undiagnosed for months. Equally troubling is the conundrum that patients with lupus tend to appear to be fine while feeling poorly, so their initial complaints are not always taken seriously.

Making an accurate diagnosis of systemic lupus can be tricky and treatment options vary. Sometimes the clinical onset of lupus is abrupt requiring prompt intervention, and other times lupus is relatively mild and remains stable for years. Most patients with lupus take a daily pill called hydroxychloroquine and some require stronger immune-modulating drugs to prevent organ damage. Prevention and monitoring are key. Watching diligently for kidney problems, miscarriage, stroke, seizure, arthritis, and cardiopulmonary issues can make all the difference. A good patient-provider relationship helps minimize these complications.

In terms of kindness, the best providers know that patients with lupus have many legitimate questions and concerns, so patience and understanding are essential. Caring for lupus means being attentive and alert while spending extra time, if necessary.

One such patient named Selina had a camera-ready smile. Come to think of it, I cannot recall seeing Selina in a bad mood despite the tough financial issues that compounded her medical problems. She worked two jobs, 40 hours full-time as a hospital nurse and part-time as a private-duty nurse totaling nearly 60 hours per week. She needed the extra money for family obligations and debt, which would have been challenging enough for most people.

I followed Selina in my office for two distinct autoimmune conditions (lupus and dermatomyositis) that were serious but manageable. Add to the mix her HIV infection and you have a rough idea of what she was facing. My staff was aware of her situation and that I was available whenever she called or asked to be seen, even in a pinch, since a mistake in judgment could be fatal. Managing immunosuppressive drugs and anti-viral medicine together is like playing tug-of-war by pulling on opposite ends of the same rope. In Selina's case, it was necessary to keep her lupus and myositis quiet, but not to the point of inviting infection—so when she felt poorly it was crucial to promptly distinguish between a flare of lupus versus an underlying infection since they're treated quite differently. Fortunately, Selina happened to be a skilled nurse with a pretty good idea of when it was time to call for help. Consequently, her hospitalizations for bacterial pneumonia and lupus pneumonitis were each quelled with proper care.

On several occasions, I had implored Selina to reduce her work hours, knowing that overwork could be harmful to her recovery—stress, exhaustion, and inadequate sleep were common culprits that could sabotage a normal immune response. After a close-call, she was agreeable and struck a deal to cut back on her second job. Her supervisor was understanding, and the paperwork required for FMLA (Family Medical Leave Act) protected her full-time job status during periods of absence. In sickness or health, Selina's work ethic was impressive; she promptly returned after illness, and she never complained. Most patients with Selina's medical problems would have sought permanent disability, but she was not one to throw in the towel. In my opinion, it's quite possible that her endurance and positive attitude have been instrumental in her success.

"The happiness of your life depends upon the quality of your thoughts."

-Marcus Aurelius

Following a hunch

There are times in medicine when spending a few extra minutes with a patient can make the difference between life and death. Mr. Kelly, a gentleman in his mid-60's, came to me with several months of bilateral knee pain. In the absence of illness or injury a non-urgent complaint like this usually turns out to be osteoarthritis. But something didn't feel right. The tenderness found on his exam extended below the knees to the shins, and the pain bothered him more at night while he was in bed. Ordinarily, the possible causes would include osteoarthritis, anserine bursitis, degenerative meniscal tears or shin splints, but the appearance of his hands had me worried.

The small joints of his fingers looked normal but the nail beds were widened over the top, a finding known in the trade as clubbing, which could be a sign of cancer or cardiopulmonary disease. With this in mind, I asked him about weight loss, smoking, cough, or a family history of cancer, and these were all negative. To follow the hunch, I requested tib/fib X-rays that showed *periostitis* (inflammation of the periosteum at the bony surface, a possible sign of cancer) and a chest X-ray that showed a mass in the left upper lobe.

After a few phone calls to expedite a workup by the oncology service, the diagnosis was confirmed and his left upper lobe (and the tumor) was resected. Within a week his knee pain went away. A single follow up in the office was brief; his knees were fine and no further arthritis care would be needed. I expressed my happiness to Mr. Kelly for his recovery with an inward sense of satisfaction that a life was saved. We shook hands and said goodbye. Later that year he sent me a Christmas card and an expression of thanks. We haven't seen each other again, yet I know we remained connected somehow.

Whether it's a small favor or a life altering event, it feels good to make a positive difference in the life of another. Every day, people pay it forward with blood donations, philanthropy, volunteer work, and other good deeds. In this way, we help ourselves while helping others, and everyone wins.

Case in point:

Let's say you're an intern at a hospital nursing station making rounds, checking lab results, typing a progress note, and working quickly because you're way behind when a family member or visitor emerges from a patient's room with that familiar quizzical look. Chances are good that lifting your head to acknowledge the visitor will distract you from your duties and set you back further. But what is your duty if not to help?

You notice that the ward clerk is apparently elsewhere, presumably a bathroom break or down the corridor helping someone else. The visitor inches closer to get your attention and you know that once you make eye-contact you will be officially involved. You hope it's an easy question like where is the restroom? Or the cafeteria? Or perhaps it's something an ancillary staff member can tend to like "my father needs a bedpan" or "my mother is due for her medicine." Whether you're a medical or clerical employee, most questions are parsed accordingly: "Do you know if my grandmother needs a prep before her procedure?" "Can you tell me if my son is getting discharged tomorrow?" There are certain situations that get everyone's attention like "The patient in room 12 is having chest pain." Or "The guy in the bed next to my brother is about to vomit." The last thing you want to do when you're at work is more work. But since you have a calling to serve and you are driven by empathy (which means it could just as easily be you or a loved one with chest pain or nausea) you rise to the occasion, set aside your personal concerns, and say the three words that everyone wants to hear: *Let me help.*

Kindred spirits

I happen to love music, especially Rock, Pop, Soul, PROG, Jazz (Oscar Peterson), Fusion (Return to Forever), Classical (Haydn), Beatles, Broadway, and anything from the 1970's. If you want to talk about music, I'm happy to oblige.

Good music reaches people on a visceral level in a way that transcends politics and other potentially divisive topics; it's a universal language that brings people together. For enthusiasts, a deep dive into the nuance of a song or a verse is satisfying even when there is disagreement—this type of sentiment was exemplified in a book titled *Pure Baseball* by first-baseman Keith Hernandez who wrote 272 pages about the pitch-by-pitch intricacies of two baseball games. His level of interest allowed him to dissect the details of each inning in a way that only a true fan could appreciate. Music lovers know what I'm talking about.

You might ask, what does music have to do with the practice of medicine? The similarity is simply this: the friendships I've developed with patients over the years have been important to me, and anything that has strengthened those bonds is important, too. Students and interns who follow me in the office might notice that I bring up the topic of current events or music or sports rather than rush into a patient's physical complaint. They quickly see there is time to bond if you make time. It's an example I've tried to set.

A music fan named Sherry comes to mind, a fifty-year-old woman whose psoriatic arthritis responded well to biologic infusions. The joints that were once painful and swollen had markedly improved and she'd since enjoyed a fairly normal life. I saw Sherry in the office a few times per year to monitor her infusions, and since she felt well most of the time with few complaints, we had extra time to talk about our favorite subject.

Sherry's favorite music was Rock, from her attire and haircut to her vibe in every way, and you could tell which bands she loved: The Dead, The Who, Zep, Tull; she'd seen them all. If she mentioned Elvis, she meant Elvis Costello. She loved the Chili Peppers, Police, ELP, YES, and Genesis. The latter PROG bands got my attention. I once bumped into Sherry at a local Kansas concert where we hugged like brother and sister. We were kindred spirits in a way that meant a lot to me. On a rare occasion, I had to evaluate a swollen joint that flared, but for the most part when I think of Sherry, I think about her love of music.

Because if feels good

A *Runner's High* is a state of euphoria that results from a rush of endorphins in those who regularly exercise. It's a major reason that distance runners bother to lace up and sweat and pant the way they do—to attain that reward—although it must be ritually practiced for the desired effect. Likewise, experienced caregivers know that helping people is not only gratifying, it actually feels good. It's a Pavlovian byproduct that becomes hardwired.

On a molecular level, acts of kindness produce comforting hormones and neurotransmitters that sustain us through the ups and downs of life. Among these tiny feel-good molecules are *oxytocin, serotonin, dopamine, endorphins, and endocannabinoids.* In real time, they produce a brief sense of satisfaction and gratification. When produced on a regular basis, the flow of these neurotransmitters promotes general happiness, social bonding, even physical comfort. It's been shown that *routine acts of kindness reduce stress hormones* such as cortisol resulting in better sleep at night and improved function during the day ahead. So, the next time you see a kind, helpful nurse at the center of a hectic clinic or busy hospital ward, and she appears to be cool as a cucumber with a ready smile, she is probably experiencing a *helper's high*.

Being there

Of the many words used to describe a quality caregiver, *being there* tops the list. *Being there* means everything to patients who reflect upon their time of need. "*Thank you for being there*"is the best praise there is.

After a lengthy hospitalization, a nurse or doctor might have forgotten about the role they played in the survival of a patient, but a sick patient will remember. Whether the heroic act was identifying a crucial warning sign or symptom, or recognizing an error before it happened, or staying late beyond the end of a shift, or responding during a tense moment, or simply holding the hand of a frightened patient—*being there* is not just a matter of punching the clock. It means taking the time to make an extra phone call to support a patient's short term disability status so they can keep their job, even if it means you must stay on hold for fifteen minutes listening to computerized music. Being there means carefully explaining difficult treatment options for the third time with kindness and understanding.

Like any medical practice, our roster includes a handful of anxious patients who need more attention than others. A talented staff knows that a phone call from a patient in this group might require more than a return call, not so much because their lives depend on it, but because *being seen* is the thing they really want. In such cases, my colleagues Drs. Rudinskaya, Spiegel, Wolinsky, Sydney Page, and Kimberly Ofoegbu were usually able to ease their minds with a cursory exam and simple reassurance. The point is, in matters of patient satisfaction, *not* being seen in a timely fashion is also remembered. And *that's* an avoidable mistake. To a worried patient, the extra effort is always appreciated.

"People will forget what you said. People will forget what you did. But people will never forget how you made them feel."

-Maya Angelou

When the chief complaint is pain

The *history of present illness* (HPI) is a part of the medical record that's been taught in medical schools for generations. The complaint of pain, for example, has seven components of the HPI that include: *location* (where does it hurt?), *onset* (how did it begin? sudden or gradual?), *duration* (when did it start? constant or intermittent?), *severity* (how much does it hurt?), *quality* (what does it feel like? burning, sharp, dull?), *associated features* (fever, nausea, numbness, weakness?), and *modifying factors* (what makes it feel better or worse?).

Buried within the HPI are valuable clues that depend on a provider's *deductive reasoning* to sort through the layers of information. *Curiosity* and *persistence* fuel a fact-finding mission that keeps a patient focused on the task at hand. The best providers give each patient an opportunity to freely talk about themselves; this is where the pearl is found in the oyster, where answers are found that might otherwise be missed. In the world of healthcare, a thoughtful listener is valuable beyond words.

A message from **Lynn about chronic pain**:

For 18 years, I have been the ping pong patient in the world of medicine. No one has been quite sure where I belong, especially because I live in the vague world of chronic pain. I have never broken a bone, never fallen off a bike. At age 42, I woke up in pain. I used to think it completely mattered where the doctor got their degree from. I used to think it was the zip code where they practiced and told me everything I needed to know. As we have come to know it, LOL.

For so long I did Google searches to find out where my physician went to school. If I was lucky enough, I found their rank in their class. Did they publish articles? Were they part of a teaching hospital? And, was there ever misconduct of any sort? More to the point, did they ever kill anyone? I became the Sherlock Holmes of doctor hopefuls. If they ticked off those boxes I was bound and determined to see them, filled with hope. Every time.

Looking for answers, I saw every traditional known specialty. When their suggestions and treatments didn't work, I sought second and third opinions. I saw John of God and the Medical Medium. I took their supplements and read their books; currently my husband enjoys them all.

Not until many years later, did I understand and appreciate the importance of kindness in a medical practice. Certainly, most of the doctors I had seen were perfectly fine. Of course, I had my share of rude. They made me cry and question myself and my reality. The experience of rude took me to dark places which in turn made me seek out more doctors. I was in a spinning wheel of modalities and ultimately on a couch for seven years. I had an agenda but inevitably we would talk about my frustration with my "condition" and the doctors I had put so much hope in. That became the focus. What a waste of time!

What we came to discover is that when I trusted the doctor, my symptoms were manageable. When I trusted all that was being done and that no one was missing anything, I came to accept my mystery diagnosis. Was I happy about it? Absolutely not. Was I more at peace with it? A solid yes.

I can recall doctors by the emotions they produce. When Dr. C in Manhattan said to me, 'you are home now, we will figure this out' my heart melted. When Dr. T stepped out of his comfort zone and realized what I really needed was to be told that every test for anything terminal had been done, my heart was more at peace. Most recently, when my new primary care physician put her arm around my very shaky body, I knew that no matter what, we were in this together. Was this all I needed? Still to be determined. But I do know that 18 years later with 60 doctors in the rearview mirror, the ones I recall are the ones that wrapped their arms around me as a whole person and understood that I was more than my numbers, my body parts, and even my pain.

A smile means everything, and eye contact means the world to patients. We need to be heard. What I have learned is that even in the slotted 15-minute time frame, it can be done. It does not take long and it won't make the next patient late. Remember when we were born and *skin to skin* contact with a parent was the first thing that mattered? Not much has changed. The same sentiment in traditional medicine includes a smile, a phone call, and maybe even a hug. Yes, kindness can change the trajectory of a patient's outcome. My advice to caregivers is, "take the time."

*

Off-duty

After hours, healthcare providers are expected to be available. Like off-duty cops who are obligated to help in any situation, caregivers are called upon for assistance or advice when least expected. Aside from being good Samaritans, we find ourselves at the behest of family and friends with questions about a new medication or their recent symptoms or their mother-in-law's operation. And we get it—people are curious about the human body and the practice of medicine—they watch TV, explore the web, and have questions. Lots of them.

So, what are we to do?

The answer is, be polite and attentive. Spend a moment, answer their questions and concerns. If you have an urge to change the subject, don't do it too hastily because that wouldn't be nice. As long as the answers are given in general terms rather than discussing any specific patient information, just as a police detective would not divulge the details of their cases, useful information can be shared without being dismissive. If you show respect for a lay person with a medical question and answer it in practical terms, it will be appreciated.

Aside from answering questions, it is a rare but important opportunity to actually help a stranger during off-hours. My own experiences in this area have been scattered over the years, including a young man who wiped out on the ski slopes suffering a neck injury with limb weakness, a sick passenger on an airline with chest pain, a neighbor whose blood pressure dropped after a bee sting, and a woman having a grand-mal seizure in a restaurant. In each situation, my assistance was appreciated and the outcome was good, however the paperwork that was required after the first two incidents (documenting the details of the occurrence, my personal contact information, and signing a bunch of disclaimers for legal purposes) was a bit unsettling.

I knew the risks of getting involved despite the Good Samaritan Law, that if things hadn't turned out well, I might have had legal exposure. For this reason, the old adage, "Is there a doctor in the house?" is not met with the same eager response as it did in years past. Regardless, caregivers should try not to worry about such things. Those with a *calling to help* must show up when it's their turn.

Organ Donors

The decision to donate a vital organ is among the kindest acts. There are two possible paths:

1) Become an organ donor upon your death

2) Be a living organ donor

Organs that can be donated *upon death* include the heart, lungs, liver, kidneys, cornea, pancreas, and small intestine—amounting to *eight lives* that can be saved by one donor! All that's needed is a signature to be registered via one of several organizations (OrganDonor.gov, CORE, UNOS). Consent can also be given prior to a risky medical procedure, otherwise permission can be granted by the family of the deceased in cases of unexpected death if the organs are viable.

Living organ donors are between the ages of 18-55 with a BMI of less than 35 (not morbidly obese) in good physical and mental health capable of informed consent. *Bone marrow* and *skin* can be donated as well as single organ (kidney) or partial organ (liver). In America, it is *illegal to get paid* to be a living organ donor, although this has been a matter of debate since there are tens of thousands awaiting organs who will die each year, and equal desire for cash among those willing to part with a body part. It's a disturbing topic that ethicists have not fully resolved. At the time of this writing, in America, by law only travel expenses, if necessary, can be reimbursed.

Among the more altruistic gestures in modern society is a *non-directed* kidney donation offered by a willing donor to a stranger with advanced kidney disease. It's a gift of life that's immeasurable. Since the first successful kidney transplant performed in Boston in 1954, ethicists have observed this rarified behavior among genetically similar family members, "unrelated" spousal donors, and complete strangers whose best genetic matches are discovered by a registry. There is no question that the readiness to serve as a living organ donor is a generous one, and parting with a healthy kidney is a choice that requires courage and kindness. For those who cannot see themselves reaching that level of self-sacrifice, becoming a registered organ donor in the event of death is the next best thing.

In my practice over the years, I've observed the organ-donor spectrum including two successful spousal kidney transplants. I've anxiously watched the clock tick down on desperately needed livers, lungs, and hearts, and I salute all who served, in life or death, as organ donors.

The word *inspiration* can mean:

1) drawing motivation from something

2) Drawing air into the lungs

But are they really different? Is there life without one or the other?

Caring for the poor

Healthcare is distributed unevenly in America. Some consider healthcare a human right and others don't, but most would agree that we don't want a population of unhealthy citizens working in restaurants, delivering packages, cleaning homes or caring for children and the elderly. Regardless, many are left uninsured and unable to get healthcare. One third of Americans seriously struggle to afford healthcare insurance, and two thirds of *uninsured* adults say they simply don't purchase health insurance because it's too expensive. Some detractors argue that universal healthcare would be overused and abused in America and therefore cost too much to taxpayers, although there is no evidence of this in other countries that provide healthcare to all.

Presently in America, there are several ways to pay for medical care:

1) Out of pocket

2) Health insurance (usually through employment, otherwise purchased via the Affordable Healthcare Act, aka Obamacare)

3) Medicare (available to American citizens over age 65, or with SS disability, kidney failure/dialysis, or ALS/Lou Gehrig's disease).

4) Medicaid (state health coverage for low-income individuals & families below the poverty line). Annual income limits for Medicaid eligibility in 2023 were appx $20,000 for single adult, $25,000 for married couples, and $30,000 for a family of four.

5) Community clinics—supported by hospitals, volunteers, charity and other funds—either free or by sliding scale.

Undocumented immigrants in America can purchase private health insurance *outside* of the federal health insurance marketplace, but it's expensive. Those below the poverty line can qualify for Medicaid regardless of immigration status, although many are cautious about coming forward and risking exposure. Undocumented immigrants over age 65 do not qualify for Medicare.

For those who need healthcare but lack insurance or federal funds, there are free clinics in most cities and towns in America where no questions are asked about immigration status, and care is mostly provided by volunteers. The support staff in such clinics is largely paid via donations and local endowments. For example, our city of Danbury, Connecticut has a 10-town catchment area of approximately 300,000 residents where insurance-poor and undocumented patients can get quality care. Our main hospital provides both primary care and subspecialty clinics on a sliding scale at minimal or no direct cost to patients. Also, the Boehringer-Ingelheim Americares Clinic provides free care to those in need within greater Danbury, and Kevin's Community Center serves the uninsured residents of Newtown, Bridgewater, and Roxbury.

In the absence of universal healthcare, it's good to know that patients in our swath of western Connecticut are largely covered regardless of financial or immigration status; it provides hope that quality healthcare is available and can be delivered to all.

For many years I supervised a weekly rheumatology clinic that primarily served low-income patients. Since part of our catchment area was considered "federally underserved" we were granted federal funds that allowed us to help patients on state assistance (Medicaid, Title XIX), insurance-poor (people with no insurance or cheap insurance), and undocumented immigrants who could not afford to see a doctor in a typical private setting. For all of them, we provided care.

Our rheumatology clinic ran on Fridays in a large multipurpose building on Main Street along with primary care and subspecialty services. Roughly one-third of our patients did not speak English, so we had translator services available in-person or on video screens. Our particular clinic cared for mostly autoimmune diseases (lupus, rheumatoid arthritis, psoriatic arthritis), managed biologic agents and disease-modifying drugs, aspirated and injected joints, treated gout, Lyme disease, osteoarthritis and other non-surgical orthopedics. The clinic was busy and the staff was great. We had multilingual receptionists up front and highly skilled nurses in the clinical area. Each session was run by an attending rheumatologist, a rotating medical resident, and a fourth-year medical student. It was a good learning environment with interesting pathology and people of various cultures.

Caring for patients with little or no money is challenging because providers rely upon resources from the state, connections from pharmaceutical companies, and favors from friends in other disciplines to get the job done. A gap in language or education requires extra attention to make sure that all directions are understood. For example: "Do NOT take this medicine if you are planning to get pregnant." "Do NOT stop taking this medicine without calling me first." "When you finish this prescription, you must go back to the pharmacy to have it REFILLED." Simple instructions are not so simple in a foreign language. Too often, patients nod their head affirmatively even if they don't quite understand. An extra moment or two to reinforce directions is worth the effort. And documentation of their understanding is key in any language.

Commonly, providers in this setting are asked to perform tedious tasks such as filling out disability forms, back-to-work letters, applications for free medication, hand-written notes to family members, and other time-consuming chores that can test the patience of a busy caregiver. But it's really all part of the job. Compliance with instructions, clinic follow-up, lab screening and other aspects of proper care is always a challenge, perhaps more so at a community clinic. At times, we'd allocate this extra work to the medical residents on service depending on their level of reliability. Rarely, the delivery of optimal care was hindered by certain financial limitations, but just as often I was gratified by the genuine thanks given by patients who were helped when they had nowhere else to turn. People who care for the poor understand what I'm getting at. It's about giving more of yourself than you get in return. For those with a calling to serve, it's a feeling of satisfaction that money can't buy.

"Be kind, for everyone you meet is fighting a hard battle."

-Socrates

When the government steps in:

The Federal *Anti-dumping law* signed by Congress in 1986 as the Emergency Medical Treatment and Labor Act (EMTALA) prohibits hospitals that receive federal funds from refusing emergency care to low-income individuals. Since then, several hospitals have been *fined for directing ambulances away from their emergency rooms,* in some cases more than 20 or 30 miles away to another facility rather than offering to treat an uninsured or undocumented patient in crisis, or an impoverished woman in labor, for financial reasons.

That we even *need* a federal law to police selfish or bigoted behavior is disappointing but not surprising. It's an example of legislating simple decency in order to expand the social safety net. Given that most hospitals already run on tight budgets and cannot afford to dispense free care to all, laws such as EMTALA help ensure that the burden is reasonably shared for the greater good. As such, federal law now states that all who seek emergency care must be *medically screened and stabilized* before being transferred to another facility, regardless of their health insurance status or their ability to pay.

Medicare, Medicaid, and SNAP

In 1965 President Lyndon B. Johnson signed Medicare and Medicaid into law as Social Security Amendments—Medicare for people over age 65 and Medicaid for low-income households that cannot afford the rising cost of healthcare and health insurance. In 2003 prescription drug benefits (Medicare part D) were added, and in 2022 the Inflation Reduction Act allowed Medicare to negotiate prices with drug companies.

The growing need for social safety nets emerged during the Great Depression of the 1930's; this led to the Social Security Act of 1935 signed into law by FDR with regular monthly benefits for those over age 65. Until then, it was not unusual for elderly impoverished citizens to live in squalor and possibly die in the streets. To counteract this, the term Social Welfare or "Relief" became law in 1935, providing funds for citizens with income below a designated poverty line. The goal was to provide *temporary* financial support until they could find work (which was scarce in the 1930's) for a more secure life. This type of assistance made a tremendous difference to poor families. Since then, the Food Stamp Act of 1964 and Supplemental Nutrition Assistance Program (SNAP) have helped offset the expense of food and assuage the plight of hunger.

The above programs—Social Security, Medicare, Medicaid, Welfare/Relief, and Food Stamps/SNAP were borne and driven by empathy and kindness for the millions of fellow citizens who need help. Taxpayers are not always happy to assist people in need, but the majority understand that it is the right thing to do, and voters have steered these important decisions in the right direction. Historical figures such as FDR and LBJ signed these landmark bills on behalf of people who might otherwise be destitute, starving, or sick, and we have all benefited to some degree.

*

Prison Medicine

One of the kindest doctors I know, Dr. Vicki Blumberg, spent the latter part of her career working in the State Prison system caring for incarcerated patients. The way she regards patients, notably sick inmates, despite the crimes they might have committed, speaks volumes about her exceptional kindness and hope for humanity. I am fully aware that some people have little sympathy for inmates, especially those who have been victims of criminal behavior. *Let them rot in jail* is a common refrain. But when you consider the scope of non-violent crimes (marijuana possession for example) that have put people behind bars in America, the degree of racial bias, the small but meaningful number of potentially innocent inmates, and the political & financial interests intent on keeping things as they are, it is clear that we need to reform and modernize this broken machine. This is her story:

Prison medicine –by **Vicki Blumberg, MD**

For nearly a decade I worked as a physician at an intake correctional facility for men where new inmates were admitted daily. After a person is arrested, he is arraigned in court where his rights are made clear to him by a judge, and he is required to enter a plea of innocent or guilty. The judge yields a great deal of power in this setting: he can grant the defendant a "promise to appear" and release him into society (to return with counsel at a later date), or for any number of complex reasons, the defendant may end up being incarcerated.

When newly admitted, an inmate with known medical problems that require ongoing treatment may experience anxiety, fear, lack of trust, and overall insecurity. Perhaps he takes medication regularly that he suddenly finds himself without, or maybe he's had no routine medical care for years. For example, newly diagnosed hypertension and diabetes are commonly revealed at an intake exam, presenting a great opportunity to make a difference in the lives of these patients.

Whether newly disenfranchised or a seasoned repeat offender, the first week of being in jail is deemed the most stressful. In men, the risk of suicide is three times higher than in the general population, with more than fifty percent successfully taking their own life within the first nine days. Tragically, for incarcerated women, the rate of suicide is *nine times* that of women in the general population. (Prison Policy Initiative 6/23/21).

Finding an ally in the building, either within the custody ranks or among the medical staff can be pivotal. A gesture as simple as putting "Mister" before the patient's last name when calling them from the waiting room (the *cage* as it is commonly referred to) can have an immediate effect of identifying me as an ally. Transgender inmates are particularly vulnerable. If the patient self-identifies as transgender, I ask them by what name they would like to be addressed. These actions have been seen by some of the correctional staff as too deferential, however I believe these courtesies, when sincerely exercised, have as their reward a relationship rooted in respect. When these roots take hold, a rapport can grow.

At an intake facility, inmates in *pretrial detention* are presumed innocent. Unless the patient has a need to divulge information, I do not ask them what their charges are. In the beginning, I remember feeling saddened by the lack of kindness and dignity with which these men were treated. I was determined to make a difference by treating them without prejudice, but my attitude and behavior were looked upon unfavorably by some of the staff—I was labeled as *naïve* or *too nice* or *enabler*, someone who could easily be manipulated. I was *criticized for some of the attributes that I had thought made me a better doctor.* One day a nurse even slapped my hand away for offering a distraught patient a tissue to wipe his nose. This startled me but I considered it a wake-up call; a warning that my degree of compassion was considered a liability.

I came to realize that the most effective place to be kind was within the confines of my small office, devoid of cameras, behind a door (albeit left ajar, as the rules dictate). I was aware that the staff was immersed in situations that made them feel unsafe at times. Personally, I felt secure while administering care for several reasons, including the rapport I'd developed with sick inmates; although after a friend of mine, a physician, was brutally attacked by an inmate whom she was caring for, I realized that safety should never be taken for granted.

I made a habit of looking inmates in the eyes while interacting with them. This was especially poignant in a correctional facility where people feel disregarded. Patients want to be seen, and they need to know that they are heard. Younger, newly-trained physicians who are technologically adept are tempted to keep their eyes on a computer screen, only to inadvertently miss out on a more meaningful, even potentially life-saving interaction. This was particularly true early on during the COVID-19 pandemic when the virus was spreading and advice from the experts shifted like a moving target. Our patients were confused, just like people everywhere, and when you add the extra layer of suspicion inherent in a correctional environment, facts were not always perceived as such. When mask-wearing was deemed mandatory for staff and inmates alike, it was all the more valuable to look directly into a person's eyes while giving info and advice to see how it was being perceived.

I believe the role of kindness in medicine cannot be overstated, though kindness towards the self has proven more elusive. After all, putting a patients' needs above our own is just part of the job, isn't it? Well, I've learned that *I cannot, and should not, want something for someone more than they want it for themselves.* It is an onerous task to try and convince a patient that it would be a better idea to take my advice than not to take it. It isn't my responsibility to twist someone's arm to do so. My job is to communicate in a language the patient understands, create an environment of cooperation, where options are presented and the patient makes his own informed decisions. The Patient's Bill of Rights applies to incarcerated patients as well as anyone. During the COVID pandemic, it became clear that an inmate's decision not to accept an offer of the vaccine, for example, or not to wear a mask at all times, had broader implications for others. Regardless, the patient has a right to refuse any non-emergent intervention. He has to live with the consequences, and so do we.

Caregivers often confuse compassion and empathy during distress. While shared happiness is certainly fine, shared suffering can be difficult. This has been an ongoing challenge for those in the helping professions, namely doctors, nurses, therapists, or anyone who directly interacts with patients. *Empathic distress* refers to a strong, aversive response to the suffering of others and a desire to withdraw from a stressful situation in order to protect oneself. *Compassion*, on the other hand, is a feeling of concern for another person's suffering, accompanied by the motivation to help. For some healthcare workers, self-kindness is manifest by a need to leave their jobs, deeming it too risky for them or their families. For others who went to work every day, during the COVID pandemic for example, we put on our personal protective equipment (PPE) and did what we were trained to do. Whether kindness, in all its forms, can fix the next serious viral pandemic is a chapter waiting to be written.

*

Don't Blame the Victim

"Life is Difficult" were the first three words of M. Scott Peck's seminal "The Road Less Traveled" written in 1978 and no less important now. In it we learn that many problems in our lives occur because of *choices* we make. In fairness, this paradigm applies mostly to matters of relationships, personal growth, and finance, but not necessarily healthcare. Yes, there are *choices* of diet, smoking, and other habits that affect our daily health, but nobody invites leukemia, scleroderma or chronic pain. The point is, not all health problems are amenable to personal control or the choices we make, and this is why caregivers withhold judgment and try to remain sympathetic to the needs of all patients.

An equally compelling book, "In the Realm of Hungry Ghosts" by Gabor Mate' explains why the lure of substance abuse is *less dictated by choice* than it may seem. While the two distinct models outlined by Peck & Mate' seem contradictory on the surface, they're actually aligned; if you read both books you will find a deeper truth that brings them closer together. Yes, we are responsible for the choices *we* make, but not for the choices that are made *for* us. It is with this in mind that doctors and other caregivers must be understanding and offer compassion, not only during cancer and illness, but when the problem is pain, substance abuse, or both.

From the mid-90's to early 2,000's doctors made the mistake of prescribing too many narcotic pain killers. Until then, Oxycodone (FDA-approved in 1976) was available by prescription but not as abused as heroin. In 1995 a time-release version called Oxycontin was approved by FDA followed by Vicodin in 1997 and the tide started to shift to prescription drug abuse. Fentanyl was first approved by FDA in 1968 but rarely prescribed until 1990 when a topical time-released patch was approved for use in chronic pain. Even then it was primarily prescribed for terminal cancer pain, however since Fentanyl is highly potent and more easily manufactured than other opiates, its black-market synthesis and import grew considerably.

As addiction and narcotic overdoses grew more rampant in the early 2,000's, prescribers and pharmaceutical companies were given stern warnings. People died and lawsuits proliferated. Patients were increasingly frustrated because fewer doctors were willing to prescribe pain medication (even for those who needed it) and the support systems in place for addicts were sorely lacking. Methadone was still available at drug treatment centers but with variable success. In 2002 the FDA approved Buprenorphine (Suboxone) to help offset opioid dependence, though not all general physicians were familiar with its proper use. Naloxone, an antidote to acute opiate intoxication, had first attained FDA approval in 1971, but patients had limited access to it. Even when Intranasal naloxone (Narcan) attained FDA approval in 2015, it was largely administered by an EMT in an ambulance setting or in the Emergency Room—otherwise it required a prescription and a trip to the pharmacy (hardly convenient during an acute overdose). Finally, in February 2023 an FDA panel voted unanimously to approve Narcan for over-the-counter purchase without a prescription.

In my career I've witnessed a wide spectrum of attitudes and behavior that govern the decisions we make for cigarette smokers, alcoholics, morbid obesity, and other common scourges. But in matters of treating pain there's a tightrope that caregivers must walk;

that is, we want to do the right thing—the compassionate thing—to help relieve suffering, but we do not want to create a new drug addict, nor do we want to perpetuate an existing addiction, or assume undue legal exposure, or feel manipulated by those with drug-seeking behavior. Balancing these issues is fraught with risk and is often deferred to a pain management specialist.

When it comes to any type of addiction, especially drugs and alcohol, it's easy to blame the victim. But if we can agree that there is a lot that we don't know about why certain people take this detour to damage their own lives and those around them—whether it's brain chemistry, emotional trauma, pain perception, nature, nurture, or whatever—at least we can agree on the healthcare side that there are counselors and caregivers who routinely set aside judgement for kindness. Whether the problem is pain or drug addiction, there is suffering that needs to be addressed. Good care begins with listening and becoming a trusted advocate. If you're not a bona fide expert in the field, pointing someone in the right direction can be very useful. Finding out which contacts and resources are available in the community for pain management, substance abuse, domestic abuse, traumatic stress, financial counseling, and other difficult circumstances are important to know *before* they're needed. A fair number of these patients have already hit rock bottom, and many feel like there is nowhere else to turn. Rather than kicking the can down the road, a committed decision to help can be gratifying beyond words.

*

Making important decisions

The term *heuristics* refers to mental shortcuts, problem-solving, and the predictability of the decision-making process. It's a fascinating subject that explains how we make choices in real time based on patterns of behavior, inherent bias, trial and error, risk tolerance, and simple instinct. These proven concepts affect everyone, including (especially) those who consider themselves immune to such things. We like to think of ourselves as unbiased, unfettered by fleeting impulses or external influences such as the opinions of other people, but how different the truth is.

The models of heuristics have been made more understandable and reproducible by scholars like Amos Tvorsky and Daniel Kahneman who have been decorated with the Nobel Prize for their work in this area. In a nutshell, the patterns of human decision-making can be broken down into basic tenants. People become overconfident when things are going well, risk-averse in the setting of perceived loss, and more selfish than they'd like to admit. If you need an example, watch any taped episode of the TV show *Deal or No Deal* and you'll see this pattern arise again and again.

Alright, so what can we do with this information beyond explaining our tendencies to choose one way or another? What does this information teach us about ourselves? And how does this pertain to providing kindness in healthcare?

In many ways we are like other primates, prone to the same primal influences (envy, greed, aggression) as our forebears. We have evolved in several important ways but not in others. The decisions faced by hunters and gatherers 10,000 years ago still resonate at the supermarket and the playground. The joys of kinship evident in family gatherings, team sports, and politics, and the pride of ascension seen in religious ceremonies and graduations are no less tribal now than before. The wants and needs of infants are baked into our DNA like the first echoes of ancient childbirth.

We think of ourselves as highly evolved and in some ways, we are but not nearly as much as our powerful weapons. And therein lies the danger: if we lack the moral authority to responsibly help each other survive, what does that say about our species and our future? Do we have a say in the fate of the world or are we merely subject to the whims of inertia?

If we could add a measure of kindness to each decision, think about the indirect benefits on geopolitics, economics, and other aspects of daily life. Even in the setting of harsh variables such as crime, poverty, natural disasters, and global conflict, our heuristics can include a measure of kindness. By doing this, we set a good example and thereby set the butterfly effect in motion.

*

When it's okay to wait

Sometimes the best decision is to do nothing. In fact, before making a medical decision, waiting is the answer to more problems than one might imagine. In our proactive, impatient society, it is assumed that action is better than inaction—and sometimes it is true; you do not want to wait during acute appendicitis or cardiac chest pain—although in certain situations *waiting* is the response that provides the best results of all.

When it comes to making an important decision, there is usually a *right thing* to do—and sometimes the right thing to do is *nothing*. The difficult part is to know when. Such is life, the nature of random acts that come and go. Like the flip of a coin, though we cannot say for sure if it will be heads or tails, we do know exactly what the *two choices* are. That is where wisdom comes in, a sign that we're not as helpless in decision making as we might think. For example, one might guess heads or tails correctly 50% of the time, but the smart money knows with 100% certainty that the answer is going to be *"heads or tails."*

Knowing each possible outcome can help ameliorate uncertainty. Likewise, if you flip the same coin 100 times, odds are good that 95% of the time the result will be heads between 40 and 60 times. That is what wisdom affords, the ability to see the bigger picture.

A similar rationale can help guide clinical decisions and reassure patients when possible. For example, the complaint of *acute low back pain* may *feel* like a problem that requires prompt intervention, even though 90% of cases will resolve with supportive measures. If there is no history of trauma, fever, weight loss, osteoporosis, cancer, or neurologic deficit, the vast majority of patients will not require MRI scanning, surgery, epidural injections, or other invasive procedures. For this reason, health insurers are reluctant to authorize an expensive MRI scan unless the patient has already had a course of physical therapy. Providers who take a careful history and perform a good neurologic exam are more likely to treat low back pain conservatively. In the absence of worsening pain or a neurologic deficit, the decision to wait is usually correct. This helps providers and physical therapists save money while comforting and reassuring patients during their recovery.

More decisions

In the medical record, the best providers document their clinical *impressions*, including a contingency plan in case they're wrong. A word or two confirming that the patient will contact the office right away if things deteriorate has become a part of the medical-legal record to protect everyone. It may sound extraneous but it gives patients a better sense of control. That's how the healing process works.

If the severity of a medical problem is uncertain and it *feels* like a decision must be made right away, it can still be approached with *restraint* rather than haste. In fact, most problems do not require an immediate resolution. Navigating this requires confidence, tact and sensitivity. Knowledge of the patient in question and a broad yet focused differential diagnosis helps to sort out the urgent nature of any medical complaint.

The decision process typically begins with *triage* by telephone or a visit to an urgent care setting. In such a situation, it's okay to defer to patients who are afraid that they are in danger. It's never a good idea to *dismiss* the concerns of a frightened patient, even if you believe that all is well. Your ability to provide reassurance and comfort will allow you to help assuage their concerns. In such a setting, ordering additional tests may not seem cost-effective in real time, but sometimes this approach serves several different functions, to get answers that will reassure a patient, or to prove that their concerns were correct after all, thus saving everyone a lot of grief. When efforts at kindness are applied to the algorithm of medical decision making, correct answers are more likely to be found.

To be sure, the decision-making process is fraught with bias and human error, because as imperfect beings we consult at least one person for each decision, and that person is ourselves. The ongoing internal monologue that accompanies our thoughts is the *voice* that answers the questions we pose to ourselves, and that *voice* can be a best friend or our worst enemy; it's the force that guides decision-making, fantasies, and basic morality. It's the very essence of perception at any given moment: I'm hungry, what should I eat? I'll get there faster if I make a right turn. Her serum creatinine rose by 0.35 even though I told her to stop Ibuprofen. The internal voice of a caregiver can make a world of difference: an unstable voice can lead to poor decisions, and a steady voice can bring a lifetime of better decisions.

A psychology professor named Paul Slovic added much to our understanding of risk analysis, decision making and judgment. As impartial as our clinical decision-making may seem, our emotions guide nearly everything we do. For example, our own likes and dislikes influence our personal beliefs about the world around us; therefore, our emotions impact the decision-making process whether we realize it or not. This is especially true in a medical environment where certainty is in short supply and providers are busy or under pressure. For this reason, healthcare providers are more susceptible (than they think) to making decisions based on gut feelings, hunches, and instincts.

Meanwhile, it's been shown that patients are more likely to participate in medical decisions that are explained to them with visceral depictions and graphic advice rather than raw data. That is, a patient's ability to *retain* medical information is heightened by a provider's ability to *reach* them on an emotional level. The connection between provider and patient is not only clinical but *emotional* too, and a successful outcome (survival, good health) is enhanced by a solid provider-patient connection.

Dr. Slovic described a phenomenon called *psychic numbing* in which one's emotional response to the suffering of an *individual* is greater than one's response to the suffering of many. It seems paradoxical but there are clear examples—though we'd like to believe that each life has equal value, a built-in defense mechanism kicks in if we're forced to acknowledge more suffering than we can humanely accept. For example, if you randomly query people about the wide-scale slaughters of people in Darfur, Myanmar, Rwanda, Cambodia, Armenia, the Holocaust, and other gross atrocities, you're likely to get a muted reaction. It's not that people don't care, but a rational person is ill-equipped to easily absorb such things, let alone explain them. In fact, the degree of compassion and concern for one person in danger begins to fade as soon as the number of victims increases *from one person to two!* In America, we hear about mass shootings all the time on television, and the reported death-toll produces no more emotion to the average viewer than if *half* the number of victims had been killed. Yet, if one child falls down a well, the nation's attention is fully invested and all eyes and ears are glued to the news until an outcome of death or rescue is fully known. People pat themselves on the back for their exhaustive concern about one child, while legislators (and the people who vote for them) remain numb to the thousands of victims of gun violence each year.

Books and TV

Ellen was involved in a serious car accident that knocked her around pretty badly and left her disabled. She was wearing a seatbelt and there were no broken bones, but she suffered nonetheless with whiplash and myofascial pain. She needed ongoing physical therapy, medical attention, prescription renewals, help with work disability, forms, letters for her attorney, and so on. On occasion, I performed paraspinal injections of bupivacaine or Sarapin that helped relieve her neck and back pain, but they lasted only a month or two.

It became clear during one of our chats that we shared a love of literary fiction and many of the same authors. It was a good doctor-patient match. Together we made progress while finding solace in Franzen, Boyne, McEwan, Roth, Towles, and more. We discovered there is no better emollient to get through an ordeal than a shared purpose; in this case, getting Ellen back to work. Our friendly discourse about talented writers was icing on the cake. One could argue that a good hairdresser or bartender does the same thing, make a connection with patrons to enhance the experience for everyone involved, and they'd be correct.

Another patient I enjoyed seeing was Christine, whose depth of knowledge about television and movies was impressive. As a TV producer, she knew the media industry inside and out including movies and entertainers, and since we were roughly the same age, our tastes overlapped quite a bit. She had a savant-like ability to recall the names of bit actors from obscure black & white sitcoms and short-run series that amused me. At the end of each office visit, I'd pimp her with questions like, "Who died first, Shirley Booth or Robert Reed? Rock Hudson or Yul Brenner?" I could never stump her.

The troubling thing about caring for Christine was that her illness had a dubious prognosis that could affect her career and shorten her life. She had scleroderma involving her lungs that made it difficult for her to walk without oxygen. The circulation to her hands had become compromised enough that her fingertips were a dusky shade of purple even with hand-warmers. When it appeared that her response to the standard of care including biologic agents and potent vasodilators was incomplete, I grew inwardly fearful. It's a scary thing when a beloved patient isn't doing well. In due course, our lighthearted discussions about TV trivia shifted to moments of cautious optimism and hand-holding.

Then one day, for reasons that were not entirely clear, Christine started to improve. Her response to treatment was confirmed, her numbers measurably better. She actually managed to turn the corner, which in scleroderma is a gift. Just a month earlier she told me that she was not afraid to die, and now we both knew her time had not yet come. We held tight to the rigorous treatment regimen while monitoring her condition with HRCT (high resolution thoracic CT scanning), right heart catheterization, and PFTs (pulmonary function tests). Having come this far, we agreed there would be no turning back.

The renewed gleam in Christine's eyes was the best thing a doctor could hope for. The last thing she asked before leaving the office that day was, "By the way, who died first, Farrah Fawcett or Michael Jackson?"

"Good question," I said. "Tell me the answer next time."

Please don't let me be misunderstood

When considering the happiness of a *provider*, it should be noted that the lack of a smile *does not* necessarily suggest a problem. Many well-adjusted caregivers, like anyone else, reserve their smiles and are fully content. It's a cultural trait in some cases and it bears reminding that the absence of overt joy is not the same as being unhappy. It is not unusual for level-headed caregivers to spend the day helping others while remaining relatively stoic. Those who do not shine with glowing energy or an effusive smile are often well-liked and highly effective. They may be truly happy without showing it. Those who don't whistle or tell jokes may demonstrate considerable compassion and provide kindness as well. If you are one of these phlegmatic souls, take heart, you are not alone. Many introverted caregivers manage to get through the day without falling apart.

Besides, it isn't helpful to smile if you don't feel like it. Maybe you didn't get much sleep because a colicky baby kept you up half the night, or your noisy neighbor is at it again, or your spouse's CPAP machine sounds like a vacuum cleaner. Whatever the reason, a carefree smile is not always available at a moment's notice. Your patients have no idea that you started the day with a flat tire, all they know is it's *their* turn to tell you about *their* troubles so you can make *them* feel better. It's a reminder that in healthcare it's not about you, which is okay because you're a professional and you understand. You are fully able to set aside your personal issues for the good of your patients. You offer kindness even when you don't feel particularly kind, and strangely enough, doing so can actually lift your mood.

It bears repeating that your ability to demonstrate kindness, even when you are not at your best, can help you get through a difficult time. It's a self-fulfilling thing. It is also part of being a professional, another reason that the calling to service is good for everyone.

That Smell

There are certain topics that healthcare professionals rarely discuss, even amongst themselves—the distinct smell of melena, a neglected diabetic foot ulcer, the metallic breath of cachexia, the acrid smell of a corpse after a failed code, the sour contents of a nasogastric tube, the fetid tonsils of strep throat, and many more. Like a bomb-sniffing dog, an experienced caregiver can recognize these smells; they reside indelibly inside our nostrils like an olfactory scrapbook. Each smell is stored for future reference to help trigger a hunch about a diagnosis.

During Medical School, I joined a group of classmates on a field trip to the coroner's office in Manhattan where I observed my first autopsy. I remember the smells emanating from a young male who had died of an overdose the night before, the dank odor of his pale skin, the bitterness of half-digested white pills inside his stomach, and the striking contents of his bowel. In the years that followed, I learned to recognize the subtle odors of diabetic ketoacidosis, alcoholism, second-hand smoke, poor dental hygiene, and other alterations of lifestyle that provide clues about one's general health. The nose is a specialized tool that is useful to caregivers as long as we do not pass judgment. We are only there to help.

Setting a good example

Question: are providers of healthcare expected to be examples of good health? The answer is yes, or at least we should try. Can a smoking doctor encourage a patient to stop smoking? Yes, she can try. Can an obese nutritionist counsel someone about weight loss? Sure, it happens all the time but the right words might not carry as much weight. The bottom line is that credibility begins with the caregiver. *"Do as I say, not as I do"* is more effective in the Marines than in healthcare where providers are questioned all the time. That's not to say each provider must be a shining example of excellent health—that would be unfair—only that a sound effort is made, which is all we can ask of others. A dentist is not expected to have perfect teeth, and a physical therapist is not expected to be an elite athlete. The only sine qua non is: don't be a hypocrite. A thoughtful caregiver will not wag a sanctimonious finger.

The notion of being a role model comes to mind. I've always been amused by celebrities and sports figures who are taken to task on social media based on their political views or social commentary, as if playing shortstop or starring in a movie qualifies them in any other way. But that's life, I suppose. Those of us in healthcare already know that the credibility we strive for in the community comes with the expectation of setting an example. We accept the added burden of trying to practice what we preach while being honest about our flaws, and we should recognize the same limitations in those we serve. We understand that some people do drugs and others are unhappy or disfigured or infected—they're not freaks. In the early 1980's, doctors and nurses were among the first to sit at the deathbeds of frightened HIV victims. By holding their hands in front of the world we set an example of kindness and tolerance. We care for clergy and criminals equally. We care for undocumented immigrants with an extra pat on the hand because we know they might be afraid of exposure. And when COVID-19 came around we set our politics aside and got to work.

Setting a good example in healthcare means demonstrating a strong work ethic, kindness, patience, reassurance, and a search for correct answers. With these attributes, caregivers forge an environment of healing and helping. We look for inspiration by observing these traits in others.

"The human being is born with an inclination toward virtue."

-Musonius Rufus

Even the best role models are flawed to some degree, which raises the question, are imperfections something to reject or rejoice? Should we accept each personality quirk as is, or are our flaws meant to challenge us in some way? Must we constantly smooth the rough edges of our lives and strive for perfection? Surely that cannot be the meaning of life.

Given the choice, it makes sense to approach the day with a modicum of self-examination and find peace. If we learn to accept the flaws of our loved ones, we can grant ourselves a bit of lenience. The Stoic maxim, "be tolerant of others and strict with yourself" recognizes the struggle to find virtue in ourselves before others, but it does not include self-flagellation.

Ideally, the goal is to accept the things we cannot change. Any twelve-stepper can tell you that; but what are the things that cannot be changed? Character. The past. The behavior of others? So many variables set the stage for a good day or a bad one, perhaps the struggle boils down to *tolerance*. We definitely have some control over that.

Special Needs

Caring for a special-needs person requires patience and fortitude. This brings to mind a woman named Paulina who was quirky in her own right and amusingly tangential, kind of like Mr. Kimball from Green Acres who took forever to explain something. If I asked Paulina a simple question like "tell me where it hurts," she would be all over the place describing everything *but* where it hurt. Still, I was especially kind to her because of the remarkable thing she did. How could I not go the extra mile for a woman who saved the life of a boy?

Her situation was this: once a week she babysat for a 12-year-old boy named Mark who was wheelchair bound with spasticity and mental disability. He communicated by grunting and was unable to perform the basic tasks of grooming, toilet, or feeding without assistance. In an unfortunate turn of events, the severity of his condition led to a family decision to place him in a state-run facility. It was heart wrenching for his parents who had four younger children and little money.

Paulina, already in her mid-sixties with her own health problems, had heard about Mark's parents' plan to give him up. Like a guardian angel, she convinced them to leave Mark with her, promising that she would take good care of him, and they agreed.

With help from her own family, Paulina made modifications to her home including a ramp and a special alcove, and she bravely took Mark under her wing. He could not be left alone for any period of time, so Paulina took him everywhere, including to her rheumatology appointments with me, and it was no easy task; folding his wheelchair and getting him in and out of her mini-van required considerable strength and patience, yet she managed to do it all.

Over the years, Mark and I had developed a friendly rapport, including a special handshake ritual in which he wouldn't let go until I did, and it was kind of funny when we were still shaking hands enthusiastically after 15 or 20 seconds. That simple routine allowed Paulina to smile for a moment. After Mark settled down with his wheelchair parked safely beside the exam table, my attention would shift entirely to Paulina.

Looking back, what piqued my curiosity most was Paulina's decision to take Mark in. It was impractical and burdensome in ten different ways, so what made her do it? Was it affection for Mark or merely a sense of responsibility? Did his special needs ignite a feeling of obligation or a calling to a higher power? Whatever the reason, I was awestruck by her sense of purpose. Paulina once said to me, "If I don't do it, who will?" She was right of course; the answer was probably *nobody*. With that, I resolved in my mind that Paulina would always get red-carpet treatment in our office. If she needed me, I would be there for her, even though she was so weird and impossible to listen to. Of far greater importance, by bringing a young boy into her home she just might have saved his life.

Akin to Mark's dilemma, it's not uncommon these days to have elderly parents who can no longer care for themselves or remain safely in their own home. Visiting Nurse services are available in most areas but may not be enough, and adult daycare is not always an option. In such cases, the prospect of placement in a nursing home hovers with its financial implications, not to mention the guilt it invokes, versus the choice of carving out a space at home with its inconveniences and daily tumult.

Ideally, the decision to welcome an elderly parent into the home of an adult child is driven by affection and a sense of responsibility, but too often these attributes are in short supply. It's become a crisis in the western world due to matters of longevity and troubling questions about the solvency of Social Security and Medicare. Who knows where this will all lead? All I know is that a woman named Paulina once made a difficult choice for a disabled boy from another family, and in the years ahead, like the boy she saved, Paulina deserves to be treated well.

The Spouse

On occasion, a patient called in from the waiting area to an exam room is joined by a spouse. The addition of a spouse can be requested for reasons that vary, such as emotional support, companionship, as a translator, or to help explain complicated directions. There are also times when the presence of a spouse is *unwanted* by the patient but happens anyway, such as an overbearing spouse (usually a husband).

It's an unsettling dynamic, usually a matter of control or less commonly abuse, and a good provider should parse this situation carefully in order to preserve a good provider-patient relationship. If you don't appease the dominant spouse, you might lose both of them, although you want to keep your best efforts focused on your patient's needs. All of this happens while watching for red flags that could implicate a problem, even a source of physical symptoms (insomnia, headache, body aches, GI issues) that can be amplified by marital discord.

I recall an imposing man standing with arms folded in my exam room answering questions for his wife as she sat meekly on the exam table. She wasn't sleeping well. She complained of an unsettled stomach and chronic pain in the neck and shoulder regions that appeared muscular on the physical exam. She had trigger points at the upper trapezius bands without neurologic deficit or signs of disc herniation. Blood tests and imaging were normal. I explained to both of them the nature of myofascial pain and how it can spread or worsen if her sleep remained fragmented, and I pointed out the safest treatment options that I felt would work best.

My patient appeared hopeful but her spouse wasn't satisfied. He wanted a more specific diagnosis and a guarantee that the treatment would be successful, otherwise he didn't want to waste their time. That's when he unfolded his arms and said, "how can you begin a treatment when you don't even know what the problem is?" It seemed like a funny question since I had already explained the diagnosis and treatment plan, or at least I thought I had. Once again, he folded his muscular forearms and said, "I run an HVAC business. If the job isn't done right, then the job isn't over. It's not like your job. In my work, we don't have problems, only solutions."

I wasn't going to compare the intricacies of a human nervous system to an air duct. I looked at his wife who said nothing. It made sense that if I wanted to help her, I had to first gain her husband's confidence, so I asked him a few innocent questions about HVAC and he was happy to respond. With each response I nodded admiringly, and by the end of the visit we were all friends. I actually learned a few things, including the impression that he posed no danger to my patient; he probably just acted that way as a defense or in a doctor's office. More importantly, his wife did well with myofascial release therapy and a short course of muscle relaxants. I was able to talk to both of them about the importance of restorative sleep and the subtle things he could do to support her, because it appeared that he actually did love her.

Another red flag among spouses is a malingering patient on the exam table requesting pain medication while the addicted spouse hovers nearby. Or a wife in denial who answers protectively for her husband in the early throes of dementia. A spouse can reveal much about what's going on at home, and an intuitive provider can help sort things out. This is especially true for patients who might be reluctant to discuss a private matter, a passive spouse victimized by an abusive partner, a financial or legal issue that can exacerbate anxiety or insomnia, or one of many sources of marital discord that can impact one's health. In each case, a caregiver who is invested in the wellbeing of *both* halves of a troubled couple can be quite helpful. To cultivate a role as a third wheel in such cases requires tact and genuine concern.

The Slow Drain

Slow drain is the precursor of job *burnout*. In healthcare, slow drain is the result of prolonged constant exposure to illness, tragedy and misery; it's the drip-drip that drains a thoughtful caregiver of personality, and it can go unnoticed for months and years.

Both burnout and slow drain are manifestations of the same culprit—chronic stress—with a subtle distinction that can be thought of as follows: *burnout* is a car stuck on the side of the road because it has run out of gas. *Slow drain* is a car that is still running on fumes while looking for a gas station. A hard-working caregiver can spend months and years—sometimes an entire career—running on fumes, yet never miss a day's work. It may not be obvious to their patients, but to friends and family the *slow drain* of a personality that used to be fun and interesting can be disturbing.

The antidote to *slow drain* is found *outside* the healthcare environment. Friendships and activities *unrelated* to medicine help us recharge our batteries, preserve our personal interests, and keep us better engaged with patients and staff. Certain cultures carve a siesta into the afternoon to accomplish this; others rely on sports and exercise to burn off steam. In any culture, outside interests and social activities are the best preventive measures.

The slow drain of personality happens to providers who work too many hours and have too few outside interests. Medical professionals should be mindful of this and remember that we do not always see it coming. Even our best friends may not be equipped to point it out to us. Surely, our patients will not tell us that we've become boring and lifeless—so I will tell you, for the sake of your patients, friends, and family, try to be interesting. The best way to accomplish this is to *be interested.* Your curiosity about the lives of others, notably your patients, will not only make you more charming and engaging in their eyes but it will keep the spark alive in your own.

Kindness in Nursing

We've all heard of the seven seas. In nursing there are six. The "six c's" of nursing are: care, compassion, courage, communication, commitment, and competence. Embedded within these attributes is *kindness.* Nurses who care for sick patients harbor kindness and patience or the whole paradigm falls apart. Without kindness, a sterile attempt to administer care would be incomplete and shunned by patients who are afraid or in pain.

Nurses play an indispensable role in the comfort and care of sick patients, as anyone who's been confined to a hospital bed will tell you. The value they bring—the *strength* they bring—is comparable to few other professions, combining clinical responsibilities, administrative skills, protective instincts, and as a liaison between patient and all others who come near. Like few others, *the word nurse itself is a noun that describes the verb.*

School nurse – by **Evanne Orlean, RN**

As far back as I can remember, I had a desire to help others. My experiences as a young woman working in medical offices and volunteering at the hospital led me to a *path in nursing.* Kindness came naturally to me. I never felt an obligation to be kind, it just seemed to be the right thing to do and provided a sense of gratification. I'd thought being kind and compassionate would lead me to work with the elderly, but as my children grew older, the opportunity arose to become a school nurse in our home town. Since the job followed the school calendar, I was able to care for my children while continuing my career. My initial role was as a *roving nurse* in several schools, caring for children from pre-K through high school. I loved being able to help children whether their problems were physical or emotional.

Later on, at the middle school where my children had attended, an opening for a school nurse was posted and I have been there ever since. My responsibilities as a school nurse include first-aid, emergencies, health visits, delivery of medications, implementing state mandates for immunizations, physicals, safety, social and mental health issues, and managing COVID-19 protocols. As a COVID-19 coordinator, I helped students and staff navigate through the pandemic. In addition to my regular duties, I was part of a team that contact-traced large numbers of students for isolation and quarantine. Many students and staff were affected by the virus and its restrictions—some days it seemed like there were not enough hours in the day. But we got through it.

Dealing with special needs students, students with anxiety issues, and students with gender and identity issues has been an additional challenge for me. I believe that any student or staff member deserves my full attention when they walk into my office. I give them space to talk about whatever it is that is on their minds, no matter how minor it may seem at first. Even on days that I am super busy, I am aware that my job requires patience and kindness. Recently, my principal told me that I have established a "culture of kindness" in my office. That's the best compliment I could have received.

Clara Barton

A key pioneer of American nursing was Clara Barton. Born in Massachusetts in 1821, she became a schoolteacher at the age of 17 and served as a self-taught nurse at age 40 during the American Civil War. While tending to wounded soldiers (both Union and Confederate), she organized the *Ladies Aid Society* that sent bandages, food and clothing to those in need, serving dangerously close to several battles.

After the war, she worked with Frederick Douglass as an activist for civil rights and with Susan B. Anthony for women's suffrage. Then in 1869, at the age of 48, she traveled to Switzerland where she was introduced to the Red Cross and invited to start an American branch, which she did. In the years that followed, bolstered by generous philanthropy, the **American Red Cross** has since responded to life threatening emergencies resulting from war, floods, fires, and hurricanes. Clara Barton's giving nature and hard work had a lasting impact on the lives of innumerable people who've never heard of her. To this day, caregivers and patients benefit from her example.

*

"I'm not Mother Teresa" is a humble disclaimer uttered by those who could never claim to serve as she did. Mary Teresa Bejaxhiu, the Albanian nun and public health nurse who died at age 87, raised the bar of kindness for everyone. While serving in Calcutta, she personally tended to babies infected with the HIV/AIDS virus as if they were her own, at a time when people were fearful of coming into contact with victims. In the years before HIV, she similarly comforted patients with Leprosy and Tuberculosis. Her behavior set a standard of good will, not only with her words (which were sparse) but with action.

Mother Teresa witnessed considerable hardship during her tenure, yet she was known to say, "Let us always meet each other with a smile." She received the Nobel Prize in 1979 for her efforts to address poverty and suffering.

The kind radiology tech

"Hi, I'm Karen," the radiology tech said through an N-95 mask. She had a nice voice and kind eyes. The MRI was routine and I wasn't worried, but I must admit it was a tight fit inside the tunnel. Until then, I'd preferred cozy spots and had never felt claustrophobic, but lying flat on my back for an hour inside the narrow tunnel, hearing myself breathe into a mask inches below a ceiling of hard plastic felt like I was buried alive.

"It's going to be loud in there," she said, holding up a pair of headphones. "Do you have a favorite music?"

This was a trick question. If the MRI results were bad, my favorite songs would forever be associated with bad news, and that would be awful. I was going to request something from *Houses of the Holy* but quickly changed my mind. "Any soft classical music would be fine," I said, hoping to be lulled into a relaxed stupor.

Like a pro, she placed an IV line without a hint of discomfort. "When the contrast goes in, you'll feel a cool flowing sensation in your arm." She explained each step of the routine with the same reassuring tone that I offered my own patients before a procedure. It was nice to know, having uttered similar instructions and explanations thousands of times, that it was not in vain.

"The test will be broken up into segments lasting between 3 and 11 minutes," she said. This minor detail didn't seem important at the time, but looking back, had she not mentioned it, or if she hadn't paused between segments to check on me, the one-hour test would have seemed interminable. Somehow, she knew it was helpful for me to know. Her subtle expressions of kindness at each break, asking me if I'm okay, telling me exactly what to expect at each stage made the experience more bearable.

Sometimes the routine chores of a caregiver are more than just routine to a concerned patient. Not only were the MRI results negative but my list of favorite songs *remained the same.* Thank you, Karen.

The Kind Hospice Aide

My mother's final year of Alzheimer's was a long goodbye. At the age of 77 she was neither the pretty 21-year-old secretary on Madison Avenue nor the wife and mother of three we had come to know. With a supportive husband (my father) in an assisted living apartment, my dear sister Evanne (a registered nurse) had managed to help keep Mom and Dad in their own home throughout their ordeal. Mom did not appear to suffer but her mind and body had effectively shut down without communication or movement; in the end there was no effort to eat or drink and little hope that she would recover. So, without objection by my father we made the heart-wrenching decision to pull her feeding tube and withhold any heroic measures. Her time had come.

We sat at her bedside and spoke to her, unsure if she was aware or precisely when she would die, but we managed to say what was heartfelt and necessary. My sister was loving and attentive during Mom's demise despite having a full-time job and a young family of her own, and my brother Steven and I had similar work commitments and lived 50 miles away. Finally, with Dad's approval, we made the decision to call Hospice to help ease Mom's final week at home.

A few days later, the local Hospice Care Network sent a woman named Valentina who knew exactly what to do. In every way, she was a gem. She tended to Mom's personal needs, applied body lotion, changed her diapers, gave sponge baths, and kept her comfortable. Dad slept in a separate bedroom at night while Valentina actually slept beside Mom in the same queen-sized bed. During the day while we visited, Valentina stroked Mom's hand, whispered into her ear, gently brushed her hair, and eased her passing as if she were a close family member.

How does one say thank you for such kindness? Other than regular donations to Hospice, I have been unable to answer this question, except to *pay it forward* whenever possible.

"In all things we should try to make ourselves feel as grateful as possible."

-Seneca

Gratitude

During difficult times it helps to remember that things could always be worse. That's not merely a rationalization but a reminder to be grateful. Many books have been written about the subject of *gratitude* and most of them can be condensed into a few short paragraphs. Suffice to say that feeling grateful is a *state of mind* that can be rehearsed. If I pause to recognize that I'm a lucky man—not only now, but every day—then a moment of failure or frustration will not seem so bad.

At the end of a long day, feelings of gratitude can sustain a tired caregiver. In their paper, "Practicing Kindness is the Best Medicine," Hazan & Haber reminded us that it's important to cultivate an environment of being thankful, to be liberal with praise of others, and to take a moment to thank those around you for their work. This is an easy way of generating a good feeling that has been shown to help patients recover better and faster, and helps the surrounding medical staff to feel okay about working hard. It takes just one crab to drag everyone down, so don't let it be you. Instead, be the positive force that generates smiles. Be grateful for the position you're in, because it truly is a source of admiration and importance.

In return, a patient is not obliged to express gratitude (nor should it be expected) although most patients are grateful enough. This is evident during the holiday season when cards, chocolates, wine and baked goods pile up in the office. Healthcare providers and staff don't work for tips, but we do get a lot of calories for our efforts.

As far as taking on the challenge of caring for emotionally needy patients, some providers are more available than others. It helps to remember that the most demanding patients might have already worn out their welcome elsewhere making them feel rejected and perhaps even more anxious if their complaints are not taken seriously. The bottom line is, if a needful patient needs extra time to be reassured, it's up to us to provide it.

"I did my own research..."

How should a healthcare provider respond to patients who claim to have already found their own answers online? It's a scenario that is happening more frequently with the tools available. Industrious patients have a specific diagnosis in mind or a particular treatment based on *the research* they did, and they want to be heard.

Powerful search engines and emerging AI are revealing more information than ever before, and the transparency of medical records has given patients additional information with access to lab results, imaging studies, and medical notes. A patient's online search might offer solutions that could be right or wrong but the provider's role is the same—*find the best answers and provide the best treatment available.* If doing so conflicts with a patient's preference, the best approach is to tactfully discuss the options.

The ultimate clinical decision may depend on the personalities involved—one may be more assertive than the other. I've seen providers who are too stubborn to listen to any contrarian viewpoint, and patients who are equally stubborn. It's a bad combination when inflexible personalities converge, but a showdown between such individuals happens less than one might think.

Ideally, there should be *flexibility on the part of the patient* to defer to the expert—but if an uninformed patient digs his heels in and confidently insists that he's correct, a caregiver should seize the opportunity to teach. Of course, this must be done carefully with respect.

All things being equal, if a patient poses a safe, *reasonable request* based on an online search, a provider who is open-minded can make the visit more pleasant by validating the patient's view. Doing so gives both parties an active role and a greater sense of purpose. Patients who participate in their own medical decision-making are actually more likely to comply with treatment and follow-up appointments. Who knows, maybe the provider will learn something too. It's all about building trust and making the best clinical decisions.

The Electronic Health Record

My first experience with the Electronic Health Record (EHR) was in the 1990's while teaching at a nearby Veteran's Hospital. I noticed the change right away when I walked into a room of bulky desktop computers where interns and residents were feverishly typing. Until then, computers were largely used for test results and orders, whereas progress notes were part of the handwritten record.

In the hospital setting prior to the EHR, an Attending Physician would stand in the hallway outside the exam room along with medical students, residents, and fellows discussing the patients' physical findings and treatment options. Then overnight, the new focus shifted away from each other to completing a medical note on a computer. When the EHR became more widely available on laptops and tablets, the focus of attention changed inside the exam room as well, from eye-contact to the screen.

Providers typing to fill in a template or talking into a voice-recognition microphone in front of the patient added some value to the visit, but most of all it created more professional-looking notes. The time required to document the complexity of each visit (for reimbursement purposes) and submit the corresponding billing codes before the end of the day added more pressure to the job of patient care. It's also created another barrier to the mix, another layer between provider and patient.

Happily, the EHR has improved many aspects of patient care such as the retrieval of medical information and the convenience of sharing information with colleagues, billing administrators and insurance companies. However, since insurers can more easily monitor the details of each patient encounter, and pre-authorization (permission) is required by insurers for anything expensive such as radiologic imaging and most forms of treatment, providers have quietly seen a reduced sense of autonomy, which does not bode well for career satisfaction.

Is the EHR profitable? Yes, for large institutions, although not necessarily for individual providers. In addition to purchasing EHR software with its required upgrades, more staff is needed for IT assistance, plus billing and coding coordinators, employees for pre-authorization requests by phone, and an army of administrators to manage them. Fair or not, these additional expenses are necessary if a provider wants to keep the doors open.

Like other industries that had once required person-to-person interaction (travel agents, stock brokers, sales clerks, and countless jobs that are slowly being replaced by automation) our medical care runs the risk of moving in that direction. It's not all bad—we learned this during the early COVID-19 outbreak when offices were closed and Telehealth became a feasible option to engage with our patients, monitor medications, answer questions, etc. Personally, I felt during that time that the screen was a poor substitute for an in-person visit. Much of the guesswork of a virtual two-dimensional physical exam impedes the judgment of caregivers and adds risk to the delivery of healthcare. Also, the time required to navigate the system and document each encounter has usurped the actual time spent with patients.

In medicine, the human touch is not easily replaced. The more time we spend on screens, the less time we spend with patients. It's simple as that. There are only so many hours in the work day and if the EHR is grabbing our attention, we must figure out a way to push back and spend our time where it's needed most.

One approach for physicians who struggle with the complexity of the EHR is the hiring of a "scribe." A medical scribe is a person who enters the exam room with the physician or PA and listens to everything in order to create a medical note, thereby reducing the provider's task of documenting the visit and focusing instead on the patient at hand. It's an idea that makes sense and allows the provider to move more efficiently from room to room. I shouldn't have to explain the downside of this arrangement, the presence of a stranger in the exam room listening to everything, including personal information that might be too embarrassing to share, and the added expense of hiring yet another employee to compensate for the complexity of the medical record. In fairness, it's money well spent for some caregivers and not for others.

Another tactic to reduce the burden of the EHR is to have the nurses and medical assistants populate the office note with information *before* the patient is seen by the provider—everything from basic history, chief complaint, medications, allergies, family history, interval history, and more—so the provider can fill in the blanks at the end. The combined information is then folded into the final note in order to justify a visit that's suitable for billing. One can argue that stuffing the note with more information (so the provider doesn't have to do it) allows the provider to focus more on the patient, but it doesn't necessarily work out that way, nor does it improve the quality of the visit, and the reason is this: whenever specific data is presented to an attending physician by staff, students, interns or residents, the answers are limited to that data. The impressions that follow are skewed accordingly. It sounds practical because it saves time, but I assure you, something is lost.

When a provider asks pertinent questions in-person, essential clues are pursued and answers are found that might otherwise be missed. I know this as an observer of well-meaning but inexperienced medical students and interns (especially in the hospital setting) whose information is not necessarily acquired from the patient directly but from the EHR notes of their predecessors. Like playing a game of "telephone" that's prone to honest mistakes, the duplicate-chain of impressions and recommendations that follow can affect a good clinical outcome.

The bottom line is, the Electronic Health Record, like any modern data base, is there to serve us and make our lives better—but it can steal the focus away from our patients. With that in mind, we should encourage cost-effective quality medical care, accurate data capture, provider-patient rapport, attention to detail, in-person contact (if possible), sufficient time to meet our patients' needs, and the best possible clinical outcome. If the EHR (or any other new technology) can help us accomplish a fraction of that, I'm all in.

Hospital Food

The 21st century has seen an extraordinary leap of progress in hospital food services. This positive change has emerged for several reasons including a more corporate view of *patients as customers* (patient satisfaction surveys), competition among hospitals for business, a growing emphasis on quality nutrition, a more international palate, requests from employees, and an emphasis on quality nutrition.

To put things in perspective, the low-budget city hospitals that I knew as a teenage volunteer in the 1970's and later as a medical student in the 1980's put food in front of us that was barely palatable. Take my word for it, the food and smell were appalling. Fast-forward to the 21st century, hospitals have modernized with attractive bistros in the main lobby for visitors and staff, and culturally varied menus for in-patients with choices that rival nearby restaurants. The positive effect on a patient's hospital experience cannot be overstated; good food is a pleasant distraction, and healthy options are part of the path to recovery.

It begins in the kitchen with creative ideas, punctual delivery of food to patients who are stuck in their beds, and attention to special needs. A variety of options range from low-sodium, gluten-free, kosher, Spanish, cardiac, vegan, soft or puree, and many more. The budget for a typical hospital cafeteria varies considerably ($1.6 million on average to as high as $38 million at the Mayo in 2020). Some may find it strange that fees for band-aids and IV fluids are similarly accounted for, but that's modern healthcare: if it's good for the customer, it's worth the expense.

Now considered essential workers along with doctors and nurses, people with culinary pursuits can enjoy a career path in the healthcare system where they make daily contributions. There is no end to the humanitarian needs locally and across the globe that intersect with quality food services.

The Lounge

When our multi-hospital group made plans to move our section to a new office suite, I was invited to sit in on an early meeting to discuss the architectural layout. I figured the invitation was merely a courtesy since I knew very little about schematics or design, so I casually joined the others at the conference table and listened while experts delivered details about their timeline and the materials required. When it seemed that they were just about finished, I chimed in.

"What about a lounge?" I asked.

The architects and administrators looked at each other. The head planner explained that additional funding was not available for that kind of thing. She assured me that there would be enough room for a water cooler, a coffee maker, and a mini-fridge. "Employees can take a break at their desks or eat lunch off-site if they prefer, but we cannot construct a lounge with the allotted space."

They looked around to see if there were any further questions.

At the time, we had a tiny break area with four chairs, but the size of our staff had more than doubled and the demands and complexity of our work had increased as well. Suddenly the prospect of working through lunch with a sandwich in one hand and a phone in the other was looming.

"I think we can do better," I interjected. "If you ask twenty people to arrive at 7:30AM and work past 5:00PM they will need a separate space to eat away from their desks and computers."

The silence that followed was awkward. The administrators and architects hadn't expected any pushback. It might have sounded unreasonable to insist that they carve out a lounge from the available space—but they actually listened and they were able to do it.

As a matter of bureaucratic planning, a lounge may seem like a needless luxury, but I would argue that complexity of modern healthcare *requires* a space that allows a staff to unwind. Call it a lounge or whatever. It's up to the leaders of any medical office to recognize this space as a necessity, to promote job satisfaction and prevent burnout, to eat lunch together, celebrate birthdays, holidays, promotions, baby showers, and everything in-between. Now more than ever, downtime is valuable and should not be wasted. It's how we recharge our batteries. Show me an engaged, energized staff and I'll show you workplace where the job gets done.

Paying it forward

Kindness spreads easily through a healthcare setting, which explains the healing nature of one facility versus the toxic nature of another. Doctors, nurses, clerical staff, and all who participate in patient care have a stake in promoting kindness, not only for the patients but for a healthy workplace, with fewer sick days and less employee turnover.

A few years ago, I went to a Major League Baseball game with my brother and nephew at a large stadium where a free t-shirt was promoted to attendees. Before leaving for the game, I'd promised my wife that I would get her one of the colorful t-shirts unaware that there was a very limited supply. As it turned out, on the way to the stadium we hit bumper-to-bumper traffic and by the time we arrived to the gate all of the t-shirts were gone. So, I sent my wife a text with the disappointing news and a sad-face emoji.

By chance, around the fifth inning I took a walk around the stadium and saw a sign that read, "Fan Assistance" booth. I approached out of curiosity and asked the gentleman sitting there how many T-shirts had been given out.

"12,000" he said, "and they went like hotcakes."

I asked if I could purchase one and he said no because it was a one-time thing. That's what I had expected, feeling no worse than before. I casually mentioned the heavy traffic that caused us to arrive late and that my wife had admired the colorful promotion. Unexpectedly, a woman standing next to me extended her T-shirt and said, "Here, take mine."

It took a moment to process her kind gesture. My usual response was something like "no, that's okay," but this time I smiled and gently took the shirt from her. I didn't want to offend her by offering money, so I asked if there was something I could do for her in return. She shook her head, "No, just pay it forward."

It was a nice moment for both of us. In the world of medicine there is similar reciprocal energy that sustains givers and recipients of kindness. The energy is gratitude.

Paying it forward - Part two

A few months after the T-shirt incident I found myself at the same baseball stadium. Sitting to my right were my brother and his son. To my left was an elderly couple in their mid-seventies, presumably husband and wife. She sat beside me and her husband to her left. As an ardent fan, I'd been to many games over the years, and until that day I had never caught a foul ball.

During the fifth inning a visiting batter sliced a foul ball into the seats along the first base line. In an instant the ball deflected off the hands of a spectator and skipped right into my lap. I was as surprised as anyone! After a few congratulatory pats on the back from the fans around me, I passed the ball to my nephew for his inspection. He gripped the Major League baseball and rolled it around his palm before returning it to me. While I considered the notion of putting the ball back into his hands for keeps, I noticed the old lady sitting beside me holding a baseball glove.

Her husband's seat was empty. Apparently, he'd stepped away to go to the restroom or concession stand and he must have asked her to hold the glove until he got back. She mentioned that they were longtime fans and he'd brought that baseball glove to every game for more than forty years without catching a foul ball. I thought, wouldn't it be a kick if the old man returned from the restroom and his wife presented him with the foul ball? She might confess later that she didn't actually catch it with his glove, but it would still be fun to watch.

So, there I was with my nephew's eyes focused on me waiting to see if I will give him the baseball, the nice old lady with the empty baseball glove, and my instinct to keep the first foul ball I'd ever caught at a major league game. I could bring the ball home to my wife so she can share the joy of holding it, or I could bring her a hug instead and share the news about how I made somebody else happy.

Bringing out the best

Does a kind gesture by one invoke a sense of benevolence in another? Put differently, why do certain people make you feel good about yourself when others don't? I mean, you're the same person wherever you go, right? Truth be told, the answer is no; our best and worst selves are regularly drawn out by others. It's a phenomenon that goes unnoticed when we're preoccupied, but personal chemistry, good or otherwise, affects both parties.

In terms of healthcare, patients and providers have a mutual stake in creating good partnerships. A woman who comes to mind is

Mildred, a 93-year-old whom I would generously describe as grumpy and disapproving. Whenever she was brought into the treatment area, the staff would smile knowingly at one another; it seemed that nothing was good enough for poor Mildred, nothing was right in the world, and there was nothing to look forward to. Worst of all, as she liked to remind everyone, her damn arthritis made every step miserable.

Her sister Evelyn accompanied her to each visit, holding her by the elbow during the slow shuffle from the waiting area to the exam table. Their husbands had been dead for decades. Evelyn was pleasant and clearly submissive in Mildred's presence. When Evelyn died at age 91, Mildred didn't want to talk about it.

Then something new happened. When an elderly neighbor had a terminal stroke, Mildred reluctantly adopted his ten-year-old Chihuahua, a four-pound dog named Princess. And a little princess she was. In short order, a new pecking order was established. Mildred fawned over that dog to their mutual delight, preparing boiled chicken, scrambled eggs, warm milk, anything for Princess. It became clear that Mildred's crabby exterior was merely a façade. Whenever I inquired about Princess an inner light would glow and a dormant smile could not be suppressed. Mildred chuckled while describing Princess watching Lassie on TV and she marveled at her little dog's habit of barking at the mirror.

Eventually, Mildred's advanced age and limitations kept her homebound. She hired a home health aide and soon there were no more office visits. I made a house call toward the end of Mildred's life to temporarily relieve her low back pain with a pair of local injections, and in the early spring we received the news that Mildred died peacefully. Princess was placed at a dog shelter before finding a new permanent home, and the cycle continued. Moments of kindness add meaning to otherwise difficult lives.

The non-compliant lawyer

Valerie was a 45-year-old patient with aggressive rheumatoid arthritis, which did not distinguish her from most other patients in the practice, except that she was also a pro-bono attorney. The causes she had championed included struggling not-for-profits and a mix of individual hardships. I had always admired her determination and the way she protected her clients, so of course I did everything I could to keep her arthritis under control so she could get out of bed each morning to do her good work.

But Valerie didn't make it easy. She understood everything about her condition and the treatments at our disposal. She knew that it was important to suppress the activity of inflammatory arthritis before permanent damage or disability, but her compliance was awful. It's just one of those crazy things that some patients go to the doctor to get help and for whatever reason they leave their good judgment behind.

"Valerie, did you get the medication?"

"Yes."

"Are you injecting it once per week?"

"No," she admitted, "but I promise I will."

I knew she was in pain. Her fingers and toes were grossly inflamed, which limited her ability to type on a computer, commute to court, and other things a busy lawyer does. So why on earth didn't she listen to reason? I began to wonder if the main issue keeping Valerie from benefiting from an effective treatment, if not her dubious judgment, was my lack of persuasion.

I thought, how does one get another to do something they don't want to? Why would a smart woman so driven to help others neglect herself that way? Surely her job required the gift of persuasion, but so did mine. It appeared that we were stuck. I prescribed a high-quality self-injectable biologic agent to relieve her symptoms, and she was reluctant to take it.

There was always the option of *infusion therapy* which would require a visit once per month for IV medication, a form of *forced compliance* that would allow an infusion nurse to witness the medication flowing into her veins; however, Valerie was always so busy with work I knew her attendance would become a real issue with cancellations and no-shows. I had resolved in my mind that the best treatment option for Valerie was self-administered weekly injections, but she would have to comply with them if she wanted to get better. I mean, didn't she want to get better? Was she afraid of needles? No, she insisted. Was it a rebellious thing? No. Fear of allergy? Fear of biologic medication? No and no.

And then it hit me, Valerie didn't have a compliance problem as much as I did. I'm the one who found frustration in trying to control the will of another. It was time for me to loosen up on the reins and give her some space. Unlike Valerie, I rarely pushed back to authority. Unlike her career of pro-bono law, medicine is a hierarchical profession founded on giving and taking orders. For years I'd taken direction from my superiors and now it was my turn to expect the same. But Valerie's world didn't work that way. She was a maverick, a stubborn idealist who used her intellect and energy to help others who are less fortunate, if not herself.

So, the next time I saw her I changed my strategy. I appealed to her the way one might appeal to a judge in court. In deference, I became the *careworn doctor* in need of a compliant patient lest I would fail to uphold *my oath*. I told her I'd grown frustrated with the course of her arthritis, the victim of sleepless nights, and there was only one person who could assuage my suffering. *I needed her help.* She knew it was mostly poor acting and tongue-in-cheek anguish but the message got through. She agreed to adhere to the self-injectable regimen *for my sake*, and she responded beautifully. Whether the driving force of her newfound compliance was joint pain or a random epiphany doesn't really matter, as long as she got better.

*

PART 2

Becoming a caregiver

The Calling

I was a happy eight-year-old kid with an interest in bugs and dinosaurs. The notion of a career in medicine had not yet occurred to me at the time, but I do remember a disabled boy who might have influenced my decision. It happened at Marine Park Day Camp, a publicly funded summer camp in Brooklyn long ago. Children were picked up at home and delivered by school bus each morning to the basement gym of a nearby school where we spent most of the day playing Nok-hockey, punch-ball, arts & crafts, and so on— not a bad deal when you consider the alternative of staying at home. Mind you, it was the late 1960's so there were children in our midst who were victims of Thalidomide exposure born without arms, blind and deaf children in the wake of German measles, and kids with remnants of Polio and Cerebral Palsy, all too common in those days.

One afternoon, we were lined up outside waiting for the yellow buses to take us home and I found myself standing beside a boy around the same age who appeared to be blind and deaf. A transistor radio-sized hearing aid stuck out of his front pocket with a pair of wires that twisted up to his ears. The bulky low-tech hearing aid made a humming sound. I wasn't sure if I should say something to him or if he even knew that I was there, so I stood by with quiet curiosity.

Minutes later we were directed to separate buses and that was that. It was a long bus ride home for me that day. When I arrived at the front door my mother asked how my day was, and I began to cry. Thinking something terrible had happened at camp or on the bus, she took me in her arms and tried to console me. I was at a loss to explain my frustration and the blatant unfairness cast upon that little boy. When I finally managed to describe what I had seen, my mother appeared relieved that her own child was okay. But I was not okay. To this day, I wonder if that experience affected my decision to be a doctor.

I suspect that most caregivers have stories like this, a desire to help when little can be done. In some cases, it triggers a calling to serve. I've since learned that I was not as helpless as I'd once thought. I could have said a few words to that little boy or taken him by the hand, maybe directed him onto his bus or given him a friendly pat on the back. Since then, I've done more to respond in real time, to do the right thing and avoid the burden of guilt that I felt that day. But it's not always easy. It helps to keep in mind that the simplest offering of comfort can bring relief to those who need it most.

The young volunteer

The Saturdays of my junior year in High School were spent volunteering at Coney Island Hospital where I was part of a group of high schoolers known as the *Health Careers Exploration Program*. It was an incubator for future doctors looking for hospital experience and a chance to serve. Brilliant teenagers like Amy Weiss and Beth

Feinman wore beige VNA lab coats with Red Cross pins. VNA stood for Volunteer Nurse Assistant in the hierarchy of hospital volunteers. Amy and Beth received batches of new recruits for orientation and familiarized them with their duties. We were an ambitious group of mostly 16 and 17-year-olds who'd built our resume's for college and gained valuable experience as ward clerks and VNA's. Remarkably, the more established volunteers were allowed to perform EKG's and other hands-on essential tasks for an understaffed city hospital.

In the beginning it was mostly scutwork—cleaning bedpans, removing soiled laundry, feeding elderly patients and sick children, rolling immobile patients over to check for decubitus ulcers, running samples to the lab—basically anything we were told to do. Emptying bedpans took some getting used to. The sight and smell of removing a waste-filled bedpan from between the legs of a stranger (without spilling any contents) required more than just a tactful invasion of privacy; it also required a graceful exit into the hallway to the flushing apparatus on the wall. Such movements were not taught elsewhere. It's one of the things a young provider learns when thrown into the deep end.

I remember once leaning forward too closely toward the face of a demented old man who grabbed me by the tie and yanked me an inch away from his oatmeal-dribbling mouth. His breath was awful. For an instant, his eyes filled with rage and I thought he might try to bite me. I pushed myself away and learned an important lesson that he might have been more frightened of me than the other way around. Poor guy, the following day I entered his room and found him in restraints.

We were told that volunteers were not allowed to say the words *dead or died*, only the term *expired* was permitted. The strict rules of decorum and dress code prepared us for the more important demands ahead. Looking back, my interactions with patients, listening to their stories, helping the nursing and clerical staff and finding my footing in a hectic city hospital were all valuable lessons. I wouldn't call it fun, but I knew that spending my free time as volunteer was a stepping stone to a meaningful career. For eight hours on Saturdays during a 40-week stretch, I learned how to assist caregivers and patients, observe urgent and bloody hospital situations, deal with repulsive smells, and somehow make a contribution. It was an introduction to a messy world of hierarchy, responsibility, and acts of kindness that a teenager rarely gets to witness. Some of us went on to careers in medicine and some didn't. In the end, I'm pretty sure that we all learned something useful.

"Educating the mind without educating the heart is no education at all."

-Aristotle

Nothing kind about cramming

After high school I attended the Sophie Davis School in New York City, also known as the *Biomed Program*, a combined college/medical school program developed for students who were willing to provide care to underserved communities. Situated uptown at CCNY in Harlem, the school accepted high school seniors with distinguished community service and sufficient grades to withstand the rigorous curriculum. Instead of the usual 8 years of school to get an MD (4 years of college plus 4 years of medical school) the curriculum was telescoped into 6 or 7 years. In return for agreeing to practice two years or more in a federally underserved area, New York City subsidized most of the tuition, a deal that was desirable to those of us with limited financial means. For this and other reasons, it was competitive to get in. The year I entered the Sophie Davis School over a thousand students applied for 70 spots.

One caveat upon entry to the program was a requirement that only a grade of A or B was allowed. This included anatomy, neuroanatomy, embryology, physiology, biochemistry, organic chemistry, pharmacology, biostatistics, plus undergrad courses such as psychology, philosophy, literature, history, sociology, etc. Any student with a grade less than a B was shown the exit, no exceptions, so there was considerable pressure to study and work hard.

My classmates were wicked-smart, some of the brightest people I've known (Lauren Balsanello, James Kenny, Leo Blachar), and though I should have no regrets, the truth is that Sophie Davis was not a happy place for me. It was an inner-city commuter school of cinder block classrooms, a basement of cadavers, and a heavy schedule. There was a major exam on Monday mornings, which meant giving up weekends in order to cram.

The first two years I carpooled with classmates from South Brooklyn (Mill Basin and Canarsie) during rush hour, a 90-minute ride that took us on the Interboro (now the Jackie Robinson Parkway) and the Van Wyk Expressway to the Triboro Bridge (now the RFK) across 125th Street to the West Side of Harlem. We usually parked on 129th Street and walked nine blocks to 138th along Convent Avenue in time for an 8:00AM class.

During the third year at Sophie Davis, rather than carpooling I took mass transit starting at East 66th Street in Brooklyn where I took the Command Bus to Kings Highway and picked up the D-Train into Manhattan to 145th street. The commute still took 90 minutes each way, but if I was able to find a seat on the bus or train, I could study or take a nap. In the fourth year, I moved to a small apartment in Sunnyside, Queens where my commute was shortened; I took the 7 Train into Grand Central, a quick shuttle across town to the D-Train and uptown to 145th Street. I managed to get through the entire pre-med curriculum until it was time to put on the white jacket and grab a stethoscope.

The five hospital clerkships (Med, Surg, ObGyn, Psych, and Peds) were followed by a year of senior electives that introduced me to three hospitals in Connecticut. Once the degree of MD was conferred, internship, residency and fellowship took another 5 years—a total of 12 years of education and training after high school.

If you're wondering what's the point of all this moaning, the answer is to put the years of hard work into perspective, to shed light on the bad in order to appreciate the good. Too often in medical training there is a loss of enthusiasm, but for those who survive the process there is a rise from the ashes. That's when kindness re-emerges. Ask any healthcare professional and they will tell you that hospital training is nerve racking and exhausting until it simply isn't anymore. That is when caregivers can look back and say it was all worth it. Like any boxer, musician, or figure skater, a proving ground is necessary.

The young social worker

Early on at Sophie Davis, a course known as PHMS (Program in Health, Medicine, and Society) placed each student into one of several health agencies in lower Manhattan to perform social outreach work. The agencies included Betances, which catered to Spanish-speaking clientele, The Chinatown Health Clinic, various SRO's (single-room occupancy hotels) to assess the health needs of homeless clients, and an outfit that I was assigned to called Project Ezra which served poor, elderly Jews living in the Lower East Side.

At Project Ezra I performed home visits to shut-in seniors who lived in small rent-controlled apartments. Most had few or no remaining social contacts and were in fair to poor health. As part of a group of that reached out to them, I was supervised by two preceptors, Gary Dreiblatt and Peyser Edelsack. The living conditions of these elderly patients were cramped and unhealthy. It seemed their families were either absent or no longer interested in their wellbeing. I was only 18 years old at the time with little knowledge of medicine, but I was assured that I had something to offer.

The goal was to make contact with my roster of seniors to assess their health needs. Among them were a former lifelong waitress, a widowed garment district worker, a retired actress from the Yiddish Theater, and several others. They were all warm and welcoming with plenty of stories to tell. Some were Holocaust survivors. It was a real eye-opener to witness the loneliness that hides in the heart of a vibrant city.

It became clear during these home visits that some of these isolated seniors scheduled doctor appointments as a means of social contact. In so doing, they utilized ambulances to and from specialty clinics, which was a drain on city resources. With this in mind, I gathered the data and wrote a paper titled, "The correlation of health behavior with the perception of social activity" which raised the merits of home visits by a visiting nurse or social worker rather than excessive medical office visits. The results showed that it is possible to save money while improving care. It turned out to be a useful learning experience, more than I'd realized at the time. In this case, I learned that caring for the underserved and impoverished cannot be taught in a textbook nearly as well as being immersed in it.

Kindness at the dawn of HIV

When I was a third-year medical student in New York City, HIV (Human Immunodeficiency Virus) was known as HTLV-3 (Human T-Lymphocyte Virus 3). At the time, there were two distinct groups of patients: IV drug-users uptown who shared needles and acquired the emerging virus, and gay men in the theater district and downtown infected with the same virus causing an illness called GRID or Gay-related Immune Deficiency. There were also early victims of transfused blood infected with HTLV-3 (including hemophiliacs), newborn babies of drug addicts, and random victims infected via heterosexual contact.

In July 1982, the term AIDS (Acquired Immunodeficiency Syndrome) was coined to bring together all victims of the viral infection and its sequelae such as Kaposi Sarcoma, Pneumocystis Pneumonia (PCP) and other horrible opportunistic infections (toxoplasmosis, candidiasis) that consumed people during the prime of their lives. It's hard to describe the atmosphere of the major NY hospitals filled to capacity with a new, mysterious, contagious, danger of a new virus unless you've been there. We've all been through the COVID-19 Pandemic, which was serious but different, because 99% survived COVID even before the vaccine.

In 1982, HIV was a death sentence.

As a medical student performing a sub-internship and a surgery clerkship, I rotated through two lower Manhattan hospitals, one on East 19th and one on West 12th at the heart of Greenwich Village. I remember the fateful day that scores of doctors, nurses, and support staff filed into the auditorium for a series of urgent meetings to discuss questions such as, how to handle a patient with AIDS? Do we need *disposable* gowns? If you step in a puddle of urine, can you keep your shoes? It sounds crazy now, but we really didn't know.

Was it necessary to wear gloves or masks? Well, to our surprise, the answer was no. Barrier methods were only required for sexual activity or potential exposure of blood products, not for routine contact. Still, it was unsettling, at least in the beginning. The greater risk was to protect the AIDS patients *from us*, because *they* were the ones who were dangerously immunosuppressed. Thus, reverse isolation was more commonly the rule.

In most cases, the team's medical students were dispatched to the rooms of HIV patients for routine matters such as vital signs, blood drawings, and daily progress notes. It sounds incredible but in 1983 during my sub-internship nearly every patient on the medical ward had AIDS. There were also patients in the hospital with common conditions such as CHF (congestive heart failure), stroke and COPD, but if there were 30 patients on my roster, 27 of them had AIDS, typically young to middle aged men dying from awful complications, wasting away with purple velvety skin lesions of Kaposi Sarcoma, hypoxic and coughing due to PCP pneumonia, blind and delirious with brain lesions of toxoplasmosis or lymphoma. That's what it was like.

Visitors were often afraid or absent except for the most attentive parents or lovers. Our roles as caregivers, besides pumping in antibiotics, regulating oxygen, and running codes, was to serve as a final contact to the outside world. The nurses were amazing and heroic as usual. Clergy did what they could. Kindness was in abundance, albeit limited by fear and caution. When I look back at that era, I'm astonished by the progress that's been made with new treatments that extend life, so HIV is no longer the death sentence it once was. But for a while it was scary as hell. I can testify on behalf of those who suffered and died in the 1980's with complications of AIDS that in most cases, they encountered kind, supportive healthcare professionals who did their best.

Into the deep end

My first night *on-call* as an intern was in the CCU (Critical Care Unit) where patients with heart attacks and other life-threatening cardiac events are placed on telemetry and receive one-on-one care. Having already performed a fourth-year elective in cardiology, I wasn't a complete stranger to such things; I'd graduated from Medical School a few weeks earlier and was capable of giving orders or running a code if necessary.

The strange thing for me, however, occurred at the very end of the day at around 2:00AM when bedside rounds were completed, notes were written, patients were tucked in for the night, and I had a chance to take a quick nap. But where? In the past as a medical student, I either worked through the night or I was sent home if there wasn't a random on-call bed somewhere—but as a new intern on-call for the CCU I was assigned a small room several feet from the electric sliding glass doors of the CCU.

The first thing that struck me as I approached the on-call room was its proximity to the CCU. Proximity as in: if a patient went into cardiac arrest a CCU nurse would press the fat red code button at the head of the bed and a "Code-99" would be announced throughout the hospital, and since the first doctor on the scene is responsible for running the code, that doctor would be me.

I wasn't scared but I felt the weight of responsibility hover during the first night on-call, as if everything I'd ever learned could be tested at a moment's notice. Inside the tiny on-call room were a cot, a pillow and blanket, empty wrappers and coffee cups in a wastebasket, and a night table with a black telephone that appeared loud even in silence. There were no cell phones yet, just a numerical beeper clipped to my scrubs.

I remember resting my head onto the pillow with eyes open, waiting for an emergency, fairly certain that there would be no sleep. And I was right, because within fifteen minutes there was a knock at the door. Expecting one of the CCU nurses, I found a buddy named Chris Snyder standing there, an intern on the floor-team who didn't know where to find his on-call room. He asked if he could crash with me. I told him there was only one small bed but he stepped inside anyway and said it was no problem, he could sleep on the floor. Poor

Chris must have been exhausted because within minutes he was curled up on the floor, snoring.

Once again, I found myself lying in bed, looking up at the ceiling, listening to Chris' snoring when my beeper went off and I was called downstairs to the ER. Two unstable cardiac patients had arrived, both requiring hospital admission—but there was only one spare bed in the CCU so somebody would have to be moved. I joined my resident downstairs in the ER and worked with her to get things moving quickly. After completing the essential work-ups and writing admitting orders for both patients, she sent me back upstairs to the CCU to transfer our only stable patient to the telemetry unit. By then, I saw the sun begin to rise, and I knew my first night on-call as an intern was almost over.

It's difficult to fathom how much is learned during a medical internship, the boatload of information and experience needed to get the job done. I learned that helping others in a stressful environment is unnerving at first, but with practice it gets easier. Even for caregivers who are kind at heart, comforting sick patients during periods of stress requires practice.

Lyme Disease and Angel Suarez

We think of Lyme Disease as a cause of summer flu, a bulls-eye rash, arthritis, and neurologic symptoms, but there are uncommon manifestations that are more difficult to recognize. When I was a young intern and testing for Lyme disease was relatively new, a patient named Angel Suarez was brought into the hospital for two reasons: first, he needed a course of IV antibiotics, and second, to have a permanent pacemaker removed. The pacer wire had been inserted only a few days earlier at another hospital where he'd presented with a pulse of 30 due to heart block. Three days *after* he was discharged, his doctors informed by the lab that his Lyme Disease test had turned positive, and since the heart block of Lyme Carditis is temporary and treatable with antibiotics, it was decided that the pacemaker should be removed.

In retrospect, Angel was a high-risk patient for tick-borne disease. It was early July (peak season for tick bites) and he was a line-worker for the electric company, which meant that he was constantly walking through weeds and tall brush. Unaware of the engorged tick in his groin, he was playing catch with his young daughters when he began to feel unwell. He had first chalked it up to getting older or maybe he was just out of shape, but when he grew lightheaded and could barely reach for the ball, he had to sit down. His wife, watching from the porch, knew that something was terribly wrong. She brought him inside for a cold drink, which didn't help, and when his breathing grew labored and his face turned pale, she called 911. Inside the ambulance enroute to the hospital, the EMT discovered his pulse of 30.

When the blood test returned positive and a diagnosis of Lyme Disease was made, Mr. Suarez didn't want to return to the hospital where the pacemaker was inserted, so he came to ours. The new problem, however, was the risk associated with extracting an embedded pacemaker wire without injuring him. Ordinarily, the tip of the wire is rooted inside the heart muscle with fish-hook-like efficiency, and removing it once it is anchored in place is risky. These days, a surgical procedure would be performed, but in the 1980's the standard of care was to extract the pacer wire by gently but persistently tugging on the wire until it could be dislodged. Doing so makes the heart rhythm erratic with prolonged, life-threatening runs of ventricular tachycardia—not a walk in the park, even for an experienced cardiologist.

Dr. Alexander was our attending cardiologist in the CCU; he explained the risks to Mr. Suarez with the understanding that time was of the essence: the longer we waited, the more scar tissue would form around the pacer lead, so it had to be removed post-haste. With that, the consent form was signed and Mr. Suarez was brought to the Cath-lab. As predicted, the procedure was a nail-biter; several dangerous runs of V-tach dropped his pressure and he nearly fibrillated, but ultimately the wire was successfully dislodged and removed. He remained in the hospital for a few days under observation while receiving Intravenous antibiotics to prevent any further manifestations of Lyme Disease.

As I walked past his room that evening, I saw Mr. Suarez surrounded by his wife and daughters, all four sharing the same hospital bed. They looked so happy I didn't interrupt.

The following morning just after rounds, I joined Dr. Alexander in the third-floor cafeteria, both of us satisfied and relieved that everything had gone well. I took a moment to inquire about his career choice of cardiology, the frequent uncertainty, the life and death decisions, and the rewards, too. He reflected briefly and said he loved all of it. The most important thing he said, is to first be a good *doctor.* I asked him what he meant and he said, make sure to give your patients what they want, which are the *Three A's... Availability, Affability, and Ability.* It's the formula for a rewarding career in medicine or anything else.

On to fellowship

Doctors who wish to subspecialize in medicine (cardiologist, hematologist, pulmonologist, etc.) must first complete a three-year residency in internal medicine followed by a two or three-year fellowship in a selected area of expertise. That's a lot of education piggy-backed onto an already exhaustive load, but there's no way around it. When I applied for a rheumatology fellowship at Yale University School of Medicine I did not expect to be accepted, but I was determined to try.

Being granted an interview in New Haven was the first hurdle. Several weeks later, a full day of interviews began with meeting the other fellowship candidates before splitting up into private interviews with each of the professors. I was friendly and relaxed since the process felt like a fait accompli, a formality that I believed would lead to a rejection letter. After all, fellowships are assigned by a "match" meaning the competing academic programs rank their candidates, the candidates rank the programs, and the computer spits out the results. Yale was a reach for me, or so I thought. When the envelope arrived and Yale welcomed me to train in New Haven I was thrilled. It was no small leap for a kid who came from humble beginnings. To this day I remain grateful that they took a chance on me.

If you're wondering, what does a clinical fellow do? In my case it meant two additional years of training at Yale University Hospital and the West Haven VA seeing patients on the hospital service and the outpatient clinic, preparing lectures to medical students and interns, making daily hospital rounds and morning report, presenting patients to senior attendings, learning procedures, developing research projects and other academic endeavors such as writing journal articles and a book chapter. It was a great experience that I'll never forget. The diversity of patients and pathology helped me become an expert in the field, and the quality of friends made in New Haven taught me more than medicine; they set an example of scholarship and kindness, and I've been happy to pay it forward.

Fitting in

When I arrived in New Haven as a clinical fellow, I felt awkward not so much because of my lack of medical expertise but because I wasn't sure that I belonged there. I felt like an imposter at an esteemed institution. Was I smart enough? What would I have to do to succeed? I did not know the answers to these questions. Fortunately, in the months ahead, I learned that getting along and being a team player was more important than having the right answers. The expertise came later.

That discovery was more valuable to my career than any prep school or family pedigree could provide. I suppose a certain insecurity was built-in because my people did not arrive to America on the Mayflower. Like so many interns and residents who've earned my admiration over the years, I shared the curious struggle of how to fit in to the profession of medicine. My grandparents arrived at Ellis Island around 1912. Their difficult journey and the persecution they left behind resonate within me as a source of humility. Likewise, my parents never went to college but they were smart, hard-working people. They set a good example and paved the way with a disciplined approach to an honest day's work that was more valuable than a trust fund.

What am I getting at here? The simple truth is that success can be measured in a variety of ways. I would venture to say that my late mother, a medical secretary who was neither wealthy nor college educated, was successful after all—married 52 years, raised three good kids, had six grandchildren, and achieved pretty much everything she wanted. My father went to trade school to become a repairman, never made much money but seemed happy with what he had, as far as I could tell. So, who am I to define success? In fact, if you check the data regarding career satisfaction among the various medical subspecialties, happiness does not correlate with income. It's something to think about when defining success, and a good reason to pause before judging others based on social status.

Do unto others

To caregivers in a teaching hospital, the *Golden Rule* applies not only to patient care but training young minds as well. Nursing

143

students and medical students are among the most vulnerable in the healthcare system; they work hard to stay afloat and keep up with the pace under considerable pressure, and their superiors—attendings, preceptors, residents, educators—can make or break them.

During high school, I worked as a cashier at a supermarket, a delivery boy for a florist, a salesclerk at a large department store, and later in college I spent the summer as a full-time waiter in Manhattan. When you come from a blue-collar family it's not enough to be a student, you must also pay your dues, usually at minimum wage. I spent countless hours at bus stops, subways, and the back of hot kitchens learning the ropes.

At the age of 20, I moved from Brooklyn to a small apartment in Queens to be closer to *the city* (people who live in the outer boroughs refer to Manhattan as "the city"). That summer I was out of bed before 5:00AM to get to work on time. I took the number 7 to Grand Central, then transferred to the number 6 train up Lexington Ave near Bloomingdales to a Greek Coffee shop on East 63rd called *Eat Here Now*. I had to be there before 6:00AM to serve breakfast to the regulars. Work as a full-time waiter opened my eyes to a different kind of pecking order and hierarchy outside of academia.

The following year at age 21, I worked again as a waiter but this time at formal affairs such as weddings and catered events where I observed the mistreatment of low-paid staff (mostly immigrants) by old-school bosses. In some ways being a waiter prepared me for Med School clerkships and internship because I encountered a few in the healthcare hierarchy who'd likely been hazed and abused themselves. At each rung of the ladder from cashier to intern, I experienced some form of minor mistreatment. I'm not complaining, just pointing out that in healthcare, like the military and certain corporate environments, there is an initiation process that is difficult to avoid. How you deal with the abusive rites of ascension predicts how well you will treat others someday.

In my career, I've had the opportunity to look down the ladder from the top—as a provider in a busy office, an attending at the hospital, and on faculty at a university medical school where I've been in a position to verbally or emotionally dress down young trainees—but I never did. Instead, I was kind to the most vulnerable, sensitive to the meek, and patient with those who struggled. Why? Because I remember. At the beginning of medical training the tense acuity and hectic pace of inner-city hospitals caught me off-guard. I was overwhelmed at times and questioned my own ability. Fortunately, most of my instructors were understanding. But that was not always the case.

In the 1980's before the Libby Zion rule, third-year medical students on the hospital wards worked over 100 hours per week and up to 36 consecutive hours at a stretch. Adding to that burden, a small number of residents preyed on young students at the bottom of the totem-pole with excessive demands knowing that a fresh batch of trainees would arrive every three months. I did my best to not be the weak antelope in the herd, and whatever attempts at abuse thrown my way (I will not name names) did not finish me. Later on, when I became a medical resident, I did not carry on the legacy.

Ultimately, treating others with kindness and respect starts at the top. Any provider in a position of authority has the privilege and responsibility of setting a good example.

PART 3

Healthcare Heroes and Role Models

There is no limit to the vastness of need. In every part of the world, healthcare charities have made an important difference by providing sustenance, food, medicine, and shelter to communities in need. Anonymously or not, the decision to help financially or otherwise is driven by kindness, the currency that matters most.

The *donation of time* is vital to those who need help. Volunteers for numerous causes provide sweat equity to food banks, soup kitchens, drivers, pet care, adult day care, Big Brothers/Big Sisters, community clinics, and critical missions in every corner of the globe. A comprehensive list of philanthropies in healthcare would be impressive, and I wish I could pay tribute to each organization by name and celebrate their acts of generosity, the lives they've saved, and the contributions they've made to relieve suffering. To say thank you to all who give and give repeatedly with sweat equity, enlisted service, or fund raising is hereby done: Thank you all.

Wealthy entrepreneurs are worth mentioning here; though they are often lightning rods for criticism, the majority put part of their fortunes to good use (Carnegie Foundation, Rockefeller, Koch, Soros, and others). Among the modern champions of global health have been Bill & Melinda Gates whose Foundation has attracted other generous contributors such as Warren Buffett, Michael Bloomberg, William Ackman, Mackenzie Scott, Mark Zuckerberg, and others. Their wealth and the initiatives of dedicated researchers, planners and volunteers worldwide have improved the lives of millions around the world with vital improvements in the areas of infection control (Malaria, HIV, TB, Leishmaniasis, Hepatitis), agriculture, nutrition, sanitation, family planning, educational grants, and global health.

In time, Bill Gates may be remembered as much for his efforts in global health as for software innovation. It's fair to say that *money* has been a key driving force behind the success of the Gates Foundation, but it is equally true that the willingness of wealthy people to part with their hard-earned fortunes begins with *kindness.*

"Others will remember you not by the size of your bank account but by the size of your heart."

-Warren Buffett

During the COVID-19 pandemic, the *Jack Ma Foundation* and the *Alibaba Foundation* donated billions of dollars worldwide in financial support, ventilators, facemasks, infrared thermometers, educational handbooks in 23 languages, and COVID-19 test kits. The number of lives saved by their generosity cannot be fully known; suffice to say that many people are alive today because of their kindness.

Jamsetji Tata of India (1839-1904) started a foundation that has since donated the equivalent in billions of US dollars toward better health and nutrition, with provisions for cancer care in India. During the COVID-19 pandemic, the *Tata Trust* was engaged again by providing PPE, test kits, masks, gloves, ventilators, and other equipment to those in need.

Long before COVID-19, notable American charities have included The American Kidney Fund, The Arthritis Foundation, Lupus Research Alliance, Mental Health America, and so many others. Private funds for health and research grants have been funded by The *Rockefeller Foundation, The Carnegie Foundation, The Wellcome Trust, The Howard Hughes Medical Institute,* and more. The largest publicly funded source of health research in the world is the *National Institute of Health* in Bethesda, MD. Each of these organizations has brought essential services and relief to patients and families. Their tireless efforts and those of all other legitimate philanthropic groups deserve our praise.

"Never doubt that a small group of thoughtful committed citizens can change the world; indeed, it's the only thing that ever has."

-Margaret Mead

Other Humanitarian Causes:

Save The Children began in 1919 at the end of World War I when British sisters Eglantyne Jebb & Dorothy Braxton brought attention to the starvation of children in Germany resulting from a strategic Allied Blockade. After the war, their foundation continued to feed starving children in Central Europe, Russia, and Turkey.

Still based in London, *Save The Children* receives generous philanthropic support that helps provide relief to families victimized by war, natural disasters, and poverty, with ongoing efforts toward education, healthcare, and nutrition. **UNICEF**, The United Nations Children's Emergency Fund, established in 1946 after World War II, provided immediate relief to displaced children and mothers in need of food, clothing, shelter, and healthcare. In the years that followed, their efforts expanded to include support of community clinics, adoption programs, children's rights, nutrition, and disease prevention. Volunteers, celebrity ambassadorships, private sponsorship, and generous government support have kept this essential mission afloat.

In 1982, **Operation Smile** was founded by a plastic surgeon, Dr. Willam Magee, and his wife, nurse Kathleen S. Magee, who performed cleft lip and cleft palate repair on impoverished patients in the Philippines. In the years that followed, they helped raise funds to dispatch Western-trained volunteer surgeons to countries in need of service.

In 1998, **Smile Train** was founded by Brian Mullaney and Charles Wang who parted with Operation Smile to develop a different approach—their novel charity focused instead on training local surgeons in impoverished nations to perform the cleft lip repair and other craniofacial surgeries. Since then, Smile Train has been an efficient model at getting the job done in partnership with hundreds of hospitals worldwide performing hundreds of thousands of free surgical procedures.

Humanitarian aid and free healthcare & surgery to poor nations and those in crisis has been the ongoing mission of **Mercy Ships**, a charitable organization founded in 1978 by Donald & Deyon Stephens. Since the vast majority of large cities are port cities, the advent of a floating hospital delivered to people in need made perfect sense. A nine-deck ocean liner was outfitted with three operating rooms, 40 hospital beds, X-Ray and lab facilities for the 350-member crew. Since then, many retrofitted ships and countless staff and volunteers have served all over the world. Mercy Ships is a predominantly Christian organization that treats patients free of charge without regard to religion, race, or gender. Their errands of mercy have taken them to ports in need of modern surgery, dental procedures, obstetric fistula repair, community clinic development, relief of natural disasters, and more. Its newest ship, the Global Mercy, can accommodate 640 people including crew and medical staff. Surely, they are deserving of praise and gratitude for "walking the walk" on water.

Kids with Cancer

It is grossly unfair when children are afflicted with serious hardship, but the facts don't lie. In the USA alone, children suffer each year from:

Poverty   11 million

Disability   3 million

Gunshots   8,000 (3,000 deaths)

Cancer   10,000 (1,100 deaths)

The most common childhood cancers are leukemia, lymphoma, neuroblastoma, kidney tumors, bone tumors, and germ cell tumors. Fortunately, the overall five-year survival of childhood cancer has risen above 85% which is great, and the work continues.

Among the kindest professionals in healthcare are those in the field of pediatric oncology—doctors, nurses, PA's, researchers, and support staff. They know that getting children and their families through the ordeal of cancer is an art within a science. Being skilled, honest, respectful, kind, and reassuring are important to keep everyone fully engaged.

Addressing the daily burdens of pain, nausea, blood draws, MRI scans, surgery, hair loss, travel, school absence, and the looming specter of mortality are all part of the job. Even celebrating remission must be done with caution and resolve. There is no aspect of childhood cancer care that is easy. For this reason, it is always a good time to offer a tip of the cap to these extraordinary caregivers.

St. Jude Children's Research Hospital in Memphis, TN was founded by entertainer Danny Thomas in 1962 for the purpose of treating children with cancer. It is largely funded by donations and does not charge patients or their families for care. They are a highly regarded charity with awards and achievements, namely ongoing cancer research and the survival of countless sick kids whose lives have been saved by their efforts. **Shriner's Children's** founded in 1922 has become a network of non-profit medical facilities spread across North America that treats children with physical disabilities, juvenile arthritis, orthopedic issues, spinal cord injury, burn victims and more. They provide medical care, equipment, physical therapy, and other essential needs, and their efforts are largely supported by private donations. St. Jude's and Shriner's are just the tip of the iceberg with other charitable organizations working hard to help children in need such as the **Make-a-Wish Foundation, Ronald McDonald House, March of Dimes, Children's Defense Fund**, and many more. The reason is clear: the plight of innocent children afflicted by hardship is unfair and unacceptable.

"No one has ever become poor by giving."

-Anne Frank

Doctors Without Borders

Some of us are old enough to remember the TV and magazine images of starving children from Biafra in 1971 with bloated bellies and sunken eyes. Sadly, the cause of their starvation was not only famine but a tense geopolitical conflict in Nigeria that effectively cut off the Biafran food supplies. It was a terrible shame.

Without taking sides, a group of daring French doctors and journalists decided to bring aid and comfort to the sick and starving people there; they founded "*Medecins Sans Frontieres*," which has since expanded over the years to include staff and volunteers from seventy countries. Their mission is to help victims of war, poverty, natural disasters, and endemic illness regardless of their political circumstance. The long list of human beings saved by this superb organization led to its recognition in 1999 with a Nobel Peace Prize.

The conflicts and tragedies addressed by *Doctors Without Borders* have included victims of civil wars, starvation, and illness in Sudan, Rwanda, Sierra Leone, Cambodia, Kashmir, Yemen, Kosovo, Haiti, and Ukraine. It is difficult to describe the bravery and generosity of people who electively enter dangerous terrain at high risk to themselves to serve a humanitarian need. Their behavior goes well beyond kindness.

Meals on Wheels

Free home-delivered food programs are available to the elderly, poor, and homebound communities. The highly popular *Meals on Wheels* program began in the United Kingdom during World War II and came to America in 1954 supported by government grants and private donations. Vital nutrition is brought directly to elderly shut-ins, disabled military veterans, and other high-risk groups with hot and frozen meals to offset the problem of hunger.

In some cases, food can be brought for a pet dog or cat as well. Staff and volunteers not only provide meals but offer valuable social contact and brief assurance that clients are safe at home. This crucial connection allows many frail seniors to remain in their homes independently.

It's incredible that a nation as prosperous as the USA has millions at risk of hunger, but we do, and those who support Meals on Wheels and similar services such as *Mom's Meals* and *Project Angel Heart* save lives. Donations are warmly accepted.

Feeding America

The philanthropic organization *Feeding America* was founded in 1979 by John van Hengel to address the problem of hunger. Since its inception, millions have benefited from food pantries and soup kitchens because of their support and direction. The sources of food have included unwanted surplus from grocery stores, restaurants, gardens and groves, with generous donations that have helped create hundreds of food banks nationwide. Their publicized efforts to improve the nutritional value of donated food have been successful as well, resulting in reduced levels of food insecurity across America. Partnerships with known chains such as Trader Joe's, 7-Eleven, and Target, just to name a few, have helped *Feeding America* minimize the plight of hunger in our midst. The kindness and generosity of those who donate (food or money) and volunteer to serve has been vital to the health of millions, and is greatly appreciated.

"Every noble deed is voluntary."

-Seneca

Jose Andres and World Central Kitchen

Founded in 2010 by renowned chef Jose Andres, **World Central Kitchen** addresses the worldwide humanitarian problem of hunger by providing meals in the wake of natural disasters and global conflicts. In so doing, chef Jose Andres and his legions of volunteers have fed millions. While most of us watch TV news about hurricanes, earthquakes, and devastating fires, World Central Kitchen (WCK) gets mobilized to the epicenters of these catastrophes to help in real time. At the peak of the COVID-19 pandemic, WCK provided meals to front-line workers and others affected by food insecurity. In 2022, chef Jose Andres and WCK distributed meals to war-torn border areas affected by the Russian invasion of Ukraine. The bravery of those who serve this organization deserve our ongoing recognition and generous philanthropic funding.

*

Selected champions of Kindness

Jonas Salk

In 1955, Jonas Salk developed a vaccine against polio, the viral infection responsible for paralysis and other serious neurologic disability. The work of Salk (and later the Sabin oral polio vaccine in 1961) led to the near eradication of polio. What remains striking by today's standards was Salk's decision to neither patent the vaccine nor seek financial profit from its distribution. "The vaccine belongs to the people," he insisted. His primary mission was to conquer polio around the world as quickly, affordably, and efficiently as possible.

In terms of kindness, Dr. Salk was an enigma; he had disdain for the limelight thrust upon him (and other public figures) and though he resented the ceaseless invasion of his privacy, he was described in the NY Times as a person of *great warmth and enthusiasm*. In any case, there is no argument that his legacy will always be kind of amazing.

Rebecca Lee Crumpler

During the 1850's-1860's while Florence Nightingale and Clara Barton were modernizing the practice of nursing, a young nurse named Rebecca Lee became the first black woman to gain acceptance into an American medical school, now called Upstate Medical University in Syracuse, NY. Upon her graduation, Dr. Lee practiced in Boston where she cared for poor African-American women and children. After the Civil War she briefly moved to Richmond, Virginia where she provided care to freed slaves who were denied care by white doctors.

Though she encountered intense racism, Dr. Rebecca Lee Crumpler treated all patients equally, regardless of their race or ability to pay. In 1883, she wrote and published "A Book of Medical Discourses," a two-part text that provided treatment options (including holistic care) for common scourges of the day such as TB, Cholera, and Diphtheria. Like most medical texts that are over a hundred years-old, the standards of care have changed, though still evident in her writings are a sense of humor and good-nature that are refreshing in any era. She died in 1895 with a brilliant legacy of kindness and caring.

"Wherever the art of medicine is loved, there is also a love of humanity."

-Hippocrates

Helen Keller

Born in Alabama in 1880, Helen Keller lost all sight and hearing due to a febrile illness at the age of 19 months. With the help of an extraordinary teacher and companion, Anne Sullivan, she learned to read, write, sign, communicate, and thrive. Their perseverance propelled Helen to Harvard and beyond, enabling her to write books, campaign for the disabled, and help launch the ACLU in 1920.

She was an ardent supporter of women's suffrage, birth control, the labor movement, the NAACP, and the American Foundation for the Blind. In 1964 she was decorated by LBJ with the Presidential Medal of Freedom. Among her more inspirational quotes were "Failures become victories if they make us wise-hearted," and "Although the world is full of suffering, it is also full of overcoming it." Hers was a remarkable life of achievement that touched many others. Helen Keller died in 1968 at the age of 87.

Li Wenliang

Dr. Li Wenliang was an ophthalmologist in Wuhan, China who died in February 2020 after contracting the COVID-19 virus from a patient. Just prior to his death, people in Wuhan were getting sick with an unexplained pneumonia that shared elements of SARS (severe acute respiratory syndrome) and ARDS (adult respiratory distress syndrome). At the same time, the CDC and International Society for Infectious Diseases alerted hospitals in Wuhan about a novel Corona virus that spread from a local market. To the dismay of the Chinese government there was confusion and growing concern about the cause and origin of the emerging syndrome and its implications.

While experts were trying to put the pieces of the puzzle together, Dr. Li Wenliang served as a *whistleblower* to alert the world about the new deadly virus and its association with local deaths due to SARS. He pleaded widely via social media to *take active respiratory precautions* despite warnings from Chinese police to refrain from spreading rumors and publishing untrue statements.

But Dr. Li did not remain silent; he bravely reported the truth from his hospital bed until his death at the age of 34. His efforts were recognized by the World Health Organization as heroic, and the Chinese Government acquiesced and honored Dr. Li Wenliang as a martyr in service to his country and the world.

Ibn Sina (Avicenna)

Ibn Sina, born in 980 A.D. in Uzbekistan, was a devout Muslim considered by many to be the Father of Modern Medicine. Among his celebrated works (written in Arabic and Persian) were The *Book of Healing* and The *Canon of Medicine*, influencing centuries of scholars. He raised awareness of the importance of ethics in science, good hygiene, psychology and logic. He was an intellectual at a time when reason was not in abundance.

To salute his work and memorialize his name, the *Ibn Sina Clinic* in Cleveland provides free quality healthcare to those in need, regardless of race or religion. Their motto and mission are one in the same: *"excellence in clinical care is not complete without compassion and empathy."* Similarly, the Ibn Sina Foundation supports and operates a group of quality, low-cost community clinics in Houston and Port Arthur, Texas.

Hippocrates

Best known as the author of the original Hippocratic Oath 2,500 years ago, Hippocrates proclaimed "First Do No Harm." His scientific understanding was less impressive and consistent with times, declaring that Nature was made of four elements—water, earth, wind, and fire—and that *illness* was due to an imbalance of the *four humors—blood, black bile* (melancholy), *yellow bile* (found in vomit and feces, responsible for short temper), and *phlegm* (associated with a phlegmatic or calm temperament).

More impressive were his contributions that were conceptual in nature, encouraging doctors to use *deductive reasoning*, adhere to *professional ethics*, foster *beneficence* (charity, mercy, kindness), *non-maleficence* (neither harm nor neglect), and show respect for a patient's *autonomy* (confidentiality). His ideas have stood the test of time and are largely the subject matter of this book. Hippocrates died in 380 BC at the age of 70 with a legacy of kindness and care as large as history itself.

*

Role Models

Several outstanding providers in our local community described their influences, role models, and ideas about the impact of kindness in medicine. Here is a sampling of their responses:

Rheumatologist –by **Alla Rudinskaya, MD**

A few years ago, one of my patients was admitted to the hospital with a postop complication. She called me from the surgical ICU and pleaded for help. There was not much I could do, but I made a few phone calls to the surgical attending and residents, and I stopped by the hospital to see her after office hours. When she was finally discharged, she sent me a thank you card that said, "I know in my heart I would have never made it out of the hospital alive without your help."

A similar card from a patient after her complicated neurosurgery said, "there are no words to describe how grateful I am for what you did for me during one of the worst times in my life."

And here is one more: "No matter what new symptom appeared you were always optimistic and encouraging that WE would get through it. You have helped me in so many ways that medicine alone could never do." I think the last line is the essence of what kindness does for the patient. It gives them a boost of hope and strength to fight.

It may seem that being kind to a patient is time consuming and not financially compensated, and this is true to some degree: making an extra phone call at the end of the day, asking the patient about her special needs kid or terminally ill spouse, reaching out to another specialist to expedite an appointment, all takes time—but it goes a long way for the patient and the physician as well. Building a solid, trusted relationship with the patient makes it easier to deal with issues down the road. For me, knowing that I have made a difference in someone's life is very gratifying. I think it is one of the factors that helps to reduce burnout.

I had an interesting realization at the beginning of the COVID pandemic. When we switched our patient visits to Telehealth, most of my patients chose to keep their follow up appointments, even if they did not seem necessary. Many of them were asking, "Dr. Rudinskaya, how are you doing?" They were checking up on me!

I believe the profession of *physician* has been romanticized. A physician is perceived as one who is expected to do good for his/her patients, placing the wellbeing of others above his/her own interests, a hero of some sort. I understand now that this expectation is not necessarily fair or right, but it played a role in building me as a physician. I was fortunate to learn from many great physicians in my Medical School in Tashkent and later during residency and fellowship at Downstate, NY who were not just great professionals but great human beings. Likewise, my parents were not physicians but they were great examples of kindness. I've also been very fortunate to work with you, Dave. You are not only an exceptional physician but you are compassionate and kind. It makes it easier to be kind when the people you work with share the same philosophy and principals.

*

Community Clinic Director –by William Delaney, MD

Dr. Dwyer was our family doctor when I was a kid growing up in Providence, Rhode Island. His office was not too far from our home, and although I did not go there very often, he made a big impression. We would wait in an old-school waiting room until the big French doors opened and we were brought into his office where he had a giant desk that really impressed me. He was just very warm and friendly and kind to our family of six Irish kids and to my parents. Years later, during my third year at Brown, a Family Practitioner made an impression on me with his approach to patient care. He kept index cards on each patient that included their problems and medications, and the rest he seemed to know by just taking care of them. I went with him on house calls, to the hospital, and to nursing homes. He was just kind and courteous and patients really loved and appreciated him. Later in my training, Dr. Paul Calabrese at Roger Williams Hospital was very kind and personable and he took the time to demonstrate bedside physical exam techniques. The other influences I should mention are **Dr. Joe Belsky** at Danbury Hospital, who provided kindness and compassion to patients regardless of their ability to pay—he always seemed to take extra time to those in need—and **Dr. Pat Tietjen**, who was patient and compassionate. Most of all, my parents, Joe and Jane Delaney were my first role models of kindness.

I have said this to many residents in training over the years: "active listening" demonstrates to a patient that you are really listening and hearing their complaints. Some doctors simply forget, probably due to burnout, how important active listening is. I remember **Dr. John Pezzimenti** talk about this in his work as an oncologist. He was the first teacher to recommended that I sit down at the edge of the bed when talking to a hospital patient. There are many cultures with different traditions and impressions of how a doctor-patient interaction should proceed, but I've never gone wrong by demonstrating "active listening." Likewise, I always recommend The Golden Rule—treat each patient as you would want your family member to be treated. It's very simple. Not complicated.

The impact of kindness on clinical outcomes is difficult to measure, but in my opinion, kindness matters greatly. When patients and their families appreciate the atmosphere of kindness in a doctor-patient relationship, they are more likely to take medications properly and comply with preventive healthcare.

*

Primary Care & Geriatrics – by Ginger Hannon, APRN

Dee Lawrence, APRN was my mentor during my clinical rotation as a clinical nurse specialist. It was her devotion and care for individuals that made me decide to go back to school to get my nurse practitioner certification. The way she interacted with patients in my opinion was amazing. She was focused on the entire individual and included their family when needed. I remember doing home visits with her when patients were unable to get to the office.

My father, Charles Ferguson, was hospitalized numerous times during my teenage years and into adulthood. I learned a lot about caring by observing him in such a vulnerable state, how he interacted with doctors, nurses and staff with kindness and sense of humor. I believe this had a profound effect on the kind treatment they provided to him in return. In essence, if you are kind to others, they will be kind to you. When I was a young student nurse doing my oncology rotation, a nurse named Joan Guariglia left a mark on me. I will never forget taking care of one gentleman who was dying of prostate cancer. She was busy getting him ready for his family to come in to visit. He was pretty unresponsive at the time, yet the manner in which she got him ready with me assisting was remarkable. I remember her taking his rosary beads and wrapping them between his fingers and making him so comfortable for his family's arrival. It was extremely touching and I have never forgotten that.

Later in my career, I had the pleasure of working with Dr. Casey Ott, a very busy and sought out geriatrician, who always showed compassion and caring towards his patients. He made himself available to patients and their families, made them feel important, and put his arm around their shoulders while escorting them out of the office. If they could not get to the office, he made an attempt to see them in their homes. They never felt abandoned.

My advice to any young person entering the health field is to treat each patient as though they were part of your family. What would you do if that was your mother or father sitting on that exam table? Also, don't be afraid to share your own feelings and personal experiences. I have found that patients appreciate this and like to know that they are not alone. Patients often voice anxiety over ordinary life issues, and just sitting with them for a few moments to listen and maybe hold their hand helps them feel so much better. Showing that you care also helps families make difficult decisions at the end of the life of a loved one.

*

Primary Care Internist – by **Dr. Vadim Tikhomirov**

I will tell you the story of the broken crystal goose. One of our favorite professors of surgery looked exactly like Santa Claus, except that he didn't have a long white beard. He was always friendly, always optimistic, always supportive. He did project kindness on the level of Santa Claus when he visited the patient wards with us. We had long conversations with him, our group of ten medical students and himself, always passionately trying to teach us the art of healing. He kept a small crystal goose on his table as a memorable gift from one of his patients. One day, when he was very unhappy with us, with our inability to ask a few questions, he became so enraged that he started pommeling both fists on the table. The goose flew in the air and broke into pieces. Everyone was shocked and quiet for a few minutes. And I was thinking, how kind to your patients you must be, to go to war on their behalf, trying to teach everything you know to the medical students to prevent our future mistakes. We were as poor as any medical students in any country, any time. But in a few days, a new crystal goose was standing on his table. The flow of kindness was his legacy.

I believe the business of healing begins with a *conversation* between the patient and a doctor. We call it physician-patient relationship, and *relationship* is the key word here; without such conversation we cannot function. In turn, there is mutual respect and perhaps even love—yes, I've seen that quite a few times and the truth is, over the years, we learn to love our patients more and more. They are a lot like our children, some behaving badly, some worse, but how can you stop loving your children? On a more subtle note, when you are giving your warmth to your patients, they are giving you their love and respect. They can heal your burnout and fatigue, your frustration and sense of powerlessness. They are healing you when you are healing them.

*

Palliative Care –by **JoAnn Maroto-Soltis, MD**

As a youth growing up in Danbury, CT, I was first introduced to **Dr. Marvin Prince**, who practiced both internal medicine and gastroenterology. My mother was a patient of his and I just happened to be with her during a routine follow up appointment after he had discovered a small lump in her breast. I remember sitting in the chair next to my mother on the exam table. When Dr. Prince walked into the room, he immediately embraced her with a warm hug and kindly shook my hand with the most reassuring smile. Even though we were bracing for the worse, the warmth and kindness he shared with us gave us a sense of calm and hope. He sat with us and went over what to expect and told my mother that he would be there for her every step of the way. I am sure that he has never known how much his kindness meant to us that day. That visit with my mother deeply impacted our ability to cope and take the next step forward. It will never be forgotten. Dr. Marvin Prince was one of the reasons that I knew that medicine would be my calling.

I practice Palliative Care, which is about caring for people with serious illness. For me personally, I've been extremely privileged to connect with patients when they are going through challenging times, when they and their families need a provider who can help them manage symptoms, advocate for them to their specialists, counsel them regarding treatments and provide guidance so that what is most important to them is center to their care plan. As a palliative care clinician, I am part of a team of dedicated individuals whose focus is the relief of suffering (physical, emotional, spiritual) and providing guidance. I often feel like that family doc from 100 years ago making house calls and just trying to make a difference in the moment. It is extremely humbling and rewarding.

I would remind anyone entering the field of medicine that there is nothing more important than the physician-patient relationship. It has somehow been diluted by technology and RVU's and the business of medicine. It is very sad to me. But if we embrace and cultivate that bond between patient and provider with sincerity and kindness, we can really have an impact—one encounter at a time—that can last a lifetime. I would also remind young clinicians how important it is to *touch* their patients. I have found that the ability to use touch during an encounter can be so powerful. While I am examining a patient, I always use it as an opportunity to not only gain medical information, but also to let them know thought touch that I can sense and feel their suffering. It is a way to bond in a very empathic and personal way that is unique to our profession. You can often sense a person's anxiety and fear immediately dissipate with a reassuring touch. It is also a very unique way, I believe, of expressing kindness from practitioner to patient.

I know without a doubt that kindness affects the clinical outcome. When I was first considering a career in medicine, I was introduced to Dr. Bernie Siegel who is a former oncologist/author of many amazing books, including my favorite, "Love, Medicine, and Miracles." When I first read the book, I was both inspired but very much skeptical. I did not have the experience to really understand what he was writing about in his book. Now, I am convinced and more than ever a believer in the incredible healing power that kindness, positive thinking, and love can have during sickness. It is so uplifting and inspiring to know that even when traditional medicine has nothing more to offer, that there are still opportunities to make a meaningful difference to a patient if we are open and look for them. Sometimes, just being present with a patient and really listening to where they are in their disease can be therapeutic. Also, letting patients know that you will be with them through every phase of illness provides them with a sense of empowerment and comfort—again, a unique way that our kindness as clinicians can have a very meaningful impact.

Over the last 20 years, there have been scientific studies that support the mind-body connection. I personally like to follow Dr. Joe Dispenza who has collaborated with the team of molecular researchers at UCSD to prove that there are healing biochemical changes that take place in the body by changing one's emotions. For those young physicians who have not yet had the opportunity to witness how kindness can translate into healing, I would suggest that they read this work themselves. For me personally, it is gratifying to see how far we've come in this field and I am excited for the future. Finally, there is proof to support what I have come to know in my own practice for some time, that true kindness, love, and support can change our reaction to stress and illness. It's powerful and inspiring.

*

Hospitalist –by **Janaka Periyapperuma, MD**

Back in Sri Lanka, my role model for kindness was Dr. Anula Wijesundara, a highly respected senior internist with 30+ years of clinical experience. She oversaw a busy 40-bed ward, two 50-patient clinics each week, and one day for endoscopies. Even with all these responsibilities, she spent time at the bedside of each patient on the ward (including Saturdays) with the medical team. She taught us clinical pearls, respected our opinions, and showed kindness toward the new trainees. She sat beside each patient, held their hand, listened to their worries, acknowledged their concerns, and comforted them in the most empathic way. I never saw her get annoyed at even the most demanding and unreasonable patient or family member. She was honest whenever she had to deliver bad news to a patient. She returned in the afternoon for quick follow up rounds, yet she never appeared to be in a hurry. She inquired about the wellbeing of her trainees, nursing staff, and ancillary staff; she treated everyone with dignity as a fellow human being. I was lucky to have her as the first supervising attending in my medical career, and I aspired to be like her.

Now that I am a supervising attending, it is my turn to be a good role model for students, interns and residents. I encourage them to talk to their patients and their families. I remind them to be kind and compassionate, to listen to their concerns and fears, and to inquire about their lives outside the hospital. It's not unusual to learn that your patients have interesting lives, achievements and service to society and country. I also believe that a good first impression helps to foster compliance with a quality medical plan. When you treat patients with kindness and honesty, they will have trust in you and your recommendations.

*

Global medicine –by **Majid Sadigh, MD**

The kindest and gentlest mentor who taught me and nurtured my growth was **Dr. Asghar Rastegar**, Professor of Medicine at Yale and

Chair of Medicine at the West Haven VA. His wealth of knowledge inspired me, and his insights into medicine, the arts, politics, and literature, were vast. His ability to critically evaluate medical articles and emerging ideas while considering their potential impact on patients at the bedside was uncanny. His commitment to advocating for patients and their families, and addressing social disparities and human rights was staunch. His professional manner, patience, transparency, and soft disposition left a permanent impression on me.

In the practice of medicine, amidst all the gaps in our knowledge and social disparities, *kindness is what fills the spaces between the scattered pieces of medicine.* I would suggest to those entering the field of healthcare, be a kind and considerate patient advocate, stand for human rights regardless of circumstances, and learn medicine to the best of your capacity. Do not compromise on your education; become a thoughtful and skillful practitioner because kindness can go a long way, but it cannot compensate for lack of knowledge.

Kindness does not necessarily give a patient with a terminal illness more days to live, but the days they have left will be of greater quality when a caring person is holding their hand and addressing their questions and concerns. Within the sphere of global medicine, I've observed that, even in an impoverished or severely limited setting, what exists between providers and patients in the face of resource scarcity is *ourselves* and the way we treat each other. In such a setting, the absence of modern technology does not leave us entirely helpless. We can fill that space with kindness and humanity that are gratifying for both patient and provider.

*

Infectious Diseases –by **John Stratidis, MD**

My journey leading to a fellowship in Infectious Diseases was due in large part to Dr. Wayne Campbell. He was a constant role model for me, not only as a clinician, but as a human being. His untimely passing was unfortunate for too many reasons to list, but I hope to continue his principles of care that embody the adage: "In the experience of being human, the human condition always comes first." As students transition into training and eventual practice, I would tell them to embrace the human condition. Taking care of a patient is so much bigger than the medical sciences, it's about marrying the discipline with the understanding of life and death. The human condition embraces both life and death, and we must remember they are equally important.

Within the specialty of Infectious Diseases, COVID-19 has certainly challenged our limitations, but I am proud that our field did not waiver as we fought for our patients. Kindness in the field of medicine is as important as any therapeutic because it creates a bond, a connection that the patient never feels alone. Kindness is inspiration, and often times provokes a renewed will for the patient.

*

Primary Care Internist – by **David Weinshel, MD**

Kindness was a trait cultivated by my parents through their words and actions. My father, a WWII veteran, always stressed the importance of helping others. He worked as a highly specialized CPA and demonstrated a friendly and considerate nature in his work. To me, that was the epitome of professionalism. Becoming a doctor was my mother's aspiration for ALL of her children. She always told us to

BE GOOD or we couldn't be successful. Along the way to becoming an internist, I found that an empathetic, friendly approach provided greater professional and personal contentment for me and my patients. Physicians have a duty to help patients. Kindness is intrinsic to that relationship. I frequently noticed this practice of kindness among many physicians and others in the community.

Excellence as a physician requires recognition that the patient's needs and concerns are paramount. Give patients (or anyone) a friendly smile and a little extra consideration, and paying it forward will be its own reward. I believe that kindness likely improves clinical outcomes. Communication is enhanced and patients open up when they feel they are heard and in a safe environment. Kindness provides that. Improved communication generally leads to a more complete exchange of information and a context to frame the situation. Additionally, the most certain belief I have about the effect of kindness on clinical interactions is that it reduces physician burnout and can make an otherwise stressful clinical encounter a pleasurable experience.

*

Rehab Medicine & Physiatry –by **Beth Aaronson, MD**

My approach to patient care has always included being an active listener. I listen with my ears and my heart; I try as best as I can to gauge how a patient and family member may be impacted by illness, disability, or loss of function. I try to build trust by making eye contact, repeating key distressing or salient points, and by helping patients prioritize their needs. In so doing, I believe that kindness can impact the clinical outcome. By showing active engagement and consistent positive reinforcement in care, a patient can experience optimism. Staying optimistic and having concrete self-help tools to deal with pain or loss of function is empowering. Going that extra step and being kind and concerned about a patient helps them to be more compliant with recommendations. It builds on a relationship that may extend beyond your specialty and enable them to seek care in other disciplines as needed.

For young people entering the health care field I would urge them to be *kind to themselves*. Mistakes will be made along the way. There will always be good and bad days and they need to remember they are only human. Being kind to oneself enables one to proceed with less fear and more compassion.

*

Rheumatologist – by **Mohamed Mohamed, MD**

A key influence for me was Dr. Abu, an Ob-Gyn physician who established the first urogenital fistula center in Sudan. Urogenital fistula is a devastating disease for women due to its associated morbidity. I watched Dr. Abu spend hours after medical rounds talking to these patients and alleviating their suffering. It was very rewarding to see these patients' appreciation of Dr. Abu's medical care and outstanding emotional support.

I consider the cornerstones for excellent medical care, besides applying evidence-based medicine, to include patient respect, communication skills, and empathy. A kind and empathetic physician enjoys better patient rapport, which consequently leads to better patient compliance and better outcomes. When necessary, psychological support plays an additional role in improving a patient's wellbeing.

*

Nurse Practitioner –by **Cortney Davis, APRN**

As a registered nurse, I believed that kindness was simply part of the fabric, part of the vocation of caregiving, but I didn't think much about what kindness in caregiving really meant. After working in a variety of settings, I learned that kindness meant being straightforward, giving bad news clearly but with empathy and a plan to go forward. Sometimes kindness was simply listening, not judging, not rushing a patient's story. But my most enduring lesson in kindness occurred many years ago when I, a caregiver, was suddenly a patient admitted for emergency surgery. As I waited on the gurney to be rolled into the OR, a nurse sat next to me asking the routine admission questions. Someone interrupted her and she turned to answer, but not before reaching out, placing her hand on my arm, *holding me* with a gentle pressure that said I'm still with you, *even though I have turned away.* That touch, that thread of connection at a time when I was frightened and vulnerable, taught me that kindness often resides in the simplest of gestures, in privacy, in a single shared moment between caregiver and patient.

So often I see young caregivers whose main focus is learning all there is to know about nursing or medicine. The work load is overwhelming, the hours are grueling, the demon of self-doubt is always nagging, and kindness takes a back seat. Who has time to listen to a patient's deepest fears when forms have to be completed and orders must be entered? What nurse has time to give a gentle bed bath to a dying patient when there are meds to give, shift reports to finish? Who has time for listening skills and empathy? My advice to those who are called to caregiving, before you enter a patient's room, pause for a moment at the door. *Realize* that someday you will also be a patient. *Look* at the person entrusted to your care. *Notice* the patient's surroundings. *Feel* the atmosphere in the room. *Open* your heart. Deep breath, then enter.

A caregiver's kindness may have a profound effect on a patient's clinical outcome. The gentle touch I'd referred to, that nurse's reassuring kindness when I was frightened, helped me to feel known, heard, cared for. Those gifts gave me an inner strength that surely helped me survive both surgery and recovery. I understood that my nurse, and by extension, other caregivers, truly had my best interests in mind. When we are kind to patients, whether it's firm and direct kindness demonstrated by truth telling and professional support, or tender kindness shown by a touch, a word, a smile, a shared tear, or simply human respect demonstrated by allowing patients to own their narratives—their stories—to listen both to their words and to the emotions behind the words, then the entire chemical and emotional chain of response to our kindness might grant patients strength, comfort, peace, courage, and if not cure, then healing.

*

PART 4

Sense & Self

"The best physician is also a philosopher"

-Galen (190 AD)

---

*T*he following passages include the less-talked-about *senses of the mind.* By examining and understanding ourselves and each other, the art of caring gets more personal, more effective, and arguably more enjoyable.

Sense is the ability to receive and react to stimuli. The five major senses—*Sight, Sound, Taste, Smell, and Touch*—are beneficial but not mandatory for a happy, productive life. Psychologists and philosophers have described more than 20 additional senses. In no particular order they include: Sense of Humor, Sense of Virtue, Sense of Purpose, Common Sense, Sensibility, Sensitivity, Sense of Reason,

Sense of Self, Sense of Morality, Gratitude, Confidence, Joy, Optimism, and others. Most human *senses* are inherent and may be intertwined in some way with kindness.

Sense of awareness

Awareness is a form of sentience that allows one to be in the moment, to be aware of feelings and surrounding events, to pick up social clues, or to be comfortably alone. Awareness helps medical providers connect with patients and anticipate their needs. Awareness helps us choose the best path forward, find our pleasures, our purpose, and our friends. It's part of a full life that brings richness to the mundane, ushers in events with greater curiosity, attentiveness and mindfulness.

In healthcare, awareness can bring comfort to a patient looking for answers. I recall seeing a young schoolteacher named Basha who presented with several years of chronic body aches, positional dizziness and fatigue. She had already seen several caregivers who tried but were unable to help. After reading through her exhaustive medical record, lab tests and imaging studies, I performed a detailed interview and exam and concluded that Basha's problems were both inherited and acquired; she had hypermobility and dysautonomia responsible for body aches, autonomic dysfunction, and positional lightheadedness.

I explained that her condition was manageable without prescription medication, surgery, or anything too risky or expensive. She was happy to discuss the pathophysiology of her symptoms and how commonly it affected other slender flexible young women like her. Her heightened *awareness* of the nature of her condition along with specialized physical therapy, vestibular therapy, attention to fluid status, and a holistic regimen allowed her to gain better control of her body and her life. Watching Basha thrive was gratifying for both of us.

When treating a chronic medical problem, a sense of awareness can help patients and caregivers endure. Like filling up at a gas station for the long journey ahead, small acts of kindness help keep the tank full.

Sense of self

Sense of self begins in the cradle, maybe even earlier. A baby experiences its first *external* stimulus at the light of birth and quickly learns its place in relation to others. It begins the process of separating from the mother's womb, and a sense of self emerges. The first and foremost influence at this stage of development comes from the mother, whose impact can range from attention and affection to neglect or abuse. Consequently, the infant's brain becomes hard-wired for life, and its responses to social cues will forever be impacted.

It's been shown that a baby nurtured by love is more likely to succeed in every aspect of life, although there is certainly no guarantee and there are many exceptions. Countless variables come into play as a child develops self-esteem (or not). The abundant plasticity of the young brain can affect one positively or adversely. For example, the shock of early trauma can become a constant demon, but the gift of plasticity can help one overcome a difficult start.

One could argue that the earliest sense of self begins in the fetal brain, though it's more likely (in the absence of a social frame of reference while floating around in the muffled warmth of embryonic fluid) that a sense of self in the womb is arbitrary at best. Once born, a baby suddenly finds itself among others with a frame of reference that becomes meaningful. A bombardment of influence from all sides forges a sense of self and a foundation of everything from tranquility to anxiety, courage to cowardice, good judgment to foolishness, and a myriad of traits that ultimately determine one's character.

Common Sense

Common sense is *sound, practical judgment concerning everyday matters.* With common sense comes the ability to choose wisely. There is no greater gift than the right to make decisions, a gift denied to millions due to oppression or forces beyond their control. The converse is also true: in a highly permissive society such as ours, opportunists feast on those with poor judgment who make bad decisions. PT Barnum wasn't an obstetrician but he knew exactly who was born every minute.

In January 1776, a 47-page pamphlet titled *Common Sense* was published (anonymously at first) by Thomas Paine focusing on the Colonists' most poignant societal issues just prior to the Revolutionary War. He posed questions that raised awareness and sharpened the will of proto-Americans to gain independence from the British Crown. Consistent with the era were statements of gross antisemitism and bigotry despite Paine's assertion of a new government of the people, but it was a big hit at the time. Suffice to say that America's struggle to form a more perfect union has been a work in progress.

Fast forward to the 21st century, the notion of *common sense* differs somewhat from Paine's—both by its meaning and by its *audience*— which is to say that *we the people* have changed. If so, what is happening to us? Are we different in some way? If the gift of sound, practical judgment concerning everyday matters is as precious now as it was in the past, what have we learned? Are we evolving into better, more enlightened people, or not at all? Has the passage of 250 years been enough time to demonstrate any significant distinction? Darwin would say no.

If not, are we different compared to humans from 10,000 years ago? Yes, in many ways. We are taller. We have less body hair. We are more informed. But are we better individuals? We live longer lives, but are our lives better? Absolutely, in many ways our lives are much better. If you are reading this book, chances are good that you have decent shelter, food, and health care, fewer threats lurking, and more opportunities to find happiness. That can change in the face of war or famine, but for now with modern technology at our disposal we have never been luckier. Perhaps with common sense, it's what we do with our advantages that will define us in history.

"There are few problems in life that kindness and common sense cannot make simple and manageable."

- Mary Burchell (aka: Ida Cook, 1904-1986)

---

*

Sense of Humor

The practice of medicine includes a smorgasbord of straight lines for the taking. The writers of the comedy series MASH were experts at parsing this by finding levity during wartime and balancing the seriousness of the moment with an open heart. They did not make light of a bad situation or risk the misperception of disrespect for the sick or dead; rather, they knew that a little humor helped to relieve tension and get everyone through the day.

In my practice, when I started writing this book, a patient arrived at her follow-up appointment with a tray of brownies that she had baked herself. I took the tray with thanks, unsure if she was playing a joke. Ordinarily, I would have tasted a brownie right in front of her, but we both knew that a week earlier she was in the hospital with a bout of Clostridium Dificile Diarrhea, a highly contagious bowel organism, and though she was feeling better she must have known that neither I nor anyone in the office would take a single bite.

Yet there was innocence in her eyes and the gesture was too kind to poke fun at, so I let it go. I set the tray aside and finished her routine visit in latex gloves. The look on my nurse's face as I offered her a brownie afterward was priceless. There was no punch-line, just a funny moment. During such times I thought of my father who would have known exactly what to say. He was a natural storyteller with a great sense of humor. Those of a certain age might recall a comedian named Myron Cohen and say they were alike. I wonder sometimes if being a raconteur has become a lost art or if it's a generational thing but Dad had heard them all, remembered them in detail, and delivered each one without a hitch. It was a rare gift and fun to be around.

At times, I would try to infuse some of Dad's playful behavior (whatever small part I might have inherited) with my patients. Being a working-class boy from Brooklyn, Dad's humor was irreverent so I was careful to share only the stories that were suitable for a medical exam room—no sex, religion, or politics. For example, there was *the one* about Mr. Schwartz, who had the rare distinction that he could only be fed *rectally*. His nurse was making hospital rounds on a beautiful sunny day when she opened the curtains.

"Good morning, Mr. Schwartz. Would you like oatmeal or a bran muffin for breakfast?"

"I'm not hungry," he said. "Just coffee, please."

"Cream and sugar?" she asked.

"Yes," he said.

She smiled and returned a few minutes later with a cup of coffee in one hand and a rectal tube in the other. Accustomed to the routine, Mr. Schwartz rolled over onto one side and waited. The nurse pushed the tube in place and began to pour.

He screamed, "Ahh! Ahh!"

The nurse jumped back. "I'm sorry Mr. Schwartz, is the coffee too hot?"

"No," he said. "Too *sweet.*"

*

I remember sharing the rectal tube story with a woman who was scheduled to have a colonoscopy, and without missing a beat she responded, "yeah, I heard about Mr. Schwartz, but did you ever meet his wife, Esther?"

"No, never," I said, playing along.

"Well, they'd been married for 50 years, and Mr. Schwartz had the annoying habit of leaving the toilet seat up. One evening, the zoftig Mrs. Schwartz was getting ready to shower and didn't realize that that toilet seat was up. When she sat down to pee, she sunk into the porcelain and she was hopelessly stuck in the low toilet.

Mr. Schwartz heard the yelling and rushed into the bathroom. He tried as hard as he could to pull his wife off the toilet but without any luck. He said, "I'm calling Tony."

"You can't let Tony in here. I'm naked, it's too embarrassing."

Thinking quickly, Mr. Schwartz took a prayer shawl and wrapped it around his wife's shoulders to cover her breasts. "There, how's that?"

"Better," she said, "but what about below? I'm exposed down there."

Mr. Schwartz took the yarmulke off his head and dropped it onto her lap. "There, that should take care of it." Satisfied that his wife was properly covered, he picked up the phone and called the superintendent of the building.

Ten minutes later, a burly man with a toolbox was greeted at the door by the elder Mr. Schwartz. He brought Tony directly to the bathroom where Esther sat blushing, a prayer shawl covering her breasts and a yarmulke over her groin. Saying little, Tony surveyed the situation, tipped his cap to the large woman stuck in the toilet, and returned to the bedroom.

"Well?" the old man asked.

"I have good news and bad news" Tony said with a heavy hand on Mr. Schwartz's shoulder. "Your wife I can save. But I'm afraid the rabbi's a *gonner.*"

*

Here's one more:

If your last name was *Diaper*, would you change it?

*

Playing in the mud

Uncertainty is part of everyday life. Like it or not, dealing with uncertainty requires humility, common sense, and wisdom. Sorting through a maze of doubt to *see things as they truly are* is a trait that is not inherent among humans but is painstakingly acquired via experience. It takes years of trial and error to attain a measure of common sense. Some call this wisdom.

This brings attention to the value of skepticism. Being aware of falsehoods should not be a source of disillusionment. Quite the opposite, *a skeptical mind is an intelligent one.* A skeptical mind is the champion of the scientific method. That's not to say that everything we believe should be subject to harsh scrutiny. Only the things we can measure should be held to that standard. One's beliefs can be flexible, and this is where the fun is—embracing uncertainty—the humble acceptance of ourselves and those we love in an imperfect world. It's the reason a hardened perfectionist may be unhappy despite prosperity, while children are happy playing in the mud.

It's a reminder that life in all its glory can be a messy thing. If you change the diaper of a beautiful baby, you quickly see the truth. From life's minor inconveniences to the cruelest mishaps, we hope to gain wisdom.

Mistakes vs. regrets

Mistakes and regrets are not the same thing. Mistakes, unlike accidents, do not necessarily occur by chance; a mistake can be the result of a *choice* that is made, and after a mistake the outcome of regret does not always follow. Regret may be immediate, delayed, or may not happen at all. One may not regret the *mistake*, but the *outcome* of the mistake. Or one can make a mistake with no regrets. This happens all the time. It begs the question, if there is no regret, can you call it a mistake?

This deserves a moment of consideration. We all make mistakes—that's part of being human, especially in healthcare—and we try to come to terms with those mistakes. Regret, on the other hand, may be the consequence of something that happened, or didn't happen, as the result of a mistake. A mistake can also be the absence of a decision. Ultimately, it's hard to say which is worse, the regret of an action or an inaction.

The old axiom, "I don't regret anything I've done in my life. My only regret is *not doing* the things I *haven't* done." But is this really possible? If one looks back regretfully, aren't they the same? One is a mistake by *choice of action* and the other is a *choice made by inaction*. Both are decisions that comprise a full life. Those who boast that they have no regrets because they're *happy with their current situation and therefore wouldn't change a thing* may be content but not entirely forthcoming. Truth be told, mistakes and regrets are equal parts of a full, interesting life.

Whether a mistake is *innocent* or *intentional*, the outcome may be a source of regret. Case in point, Charles misses a crucial decimal on a tax form and unknowingly saves a significant sum of money. James *intentionally* omits an item on his tax form resulting in the same amount of savings. Both errors may pass unnoticed, but James will only regret his behavior if he gets caught, which says something about his character. Charles may remain oblivious to the mistake that was made in his favor. In healthcare, mistakes are made with a heavy cost on both sides, and the *regret* that follows can be significant.

For better or worse, the pages of our lives are written with indelible ink. We cannot undo our mistakes; we can only reconcile them. That's where conscience comes in, the residue of guilt and the expression of remorse (or lack of it) that guides our attitudes and behavior. In the aftermath of a mistake, the presence or absence of regret is forged by conscience and character. For example, an absentee father may spend a lifetime making up for lost time with a grown child, and that child may, in turn, allow him or deny him the opportunity. A drunk driver may suffer the tragic consequences of her carelessness for the rest of her life, or if she's lucky enough to harm no one she may experience an epiphany – a wakeup call – or a second chance. Some may wonder if these endless permutations are doled out by divine intervention or karma or random happenstance. In any case, the choices we make are ours, and the consequences are as well.

"If anyone can prove and show to me that I think or act in error, I will gladly change it—for I seek the truth, by which no one has ever been harmed."

-Marcus Aurelius

Deception

One of the great masqueraders in society is bullshit. For this dubious honor, I find it peculiar that a bull was chosen from all other species. A bull is a dominant, regal, confident animal that is not given to deceiving *others* (though it may *be* deceived by a red cape). Why not a hyena or a baboon or a less reputable character? Unless that's exactly the point, that BS is synonymous with the red cape.

Those who possess the gift of common sense can detect BS; they see it coming a mile away. A heightened sensitivity to detecting BS is both an attribute and a curse given the boatload of BS that must be endured every day. The perpetrators of BS are dubbed "bullshit artists" as if the *artistry of deception* is a virtue, like the term *con-artist* which implies a mastery of confidence but is actually a form of sociopathic behavior. In either case, whether one is a bullshit artist or a con-artist, the antidote for (or the vaccine against) deception is *common sense*. As it turns out, common sense is at once a gift and a reward for alertness in a predatory world, a world in which man's worst enemy is no longer a saber-toothed tiger, but each other. One must be mindful and vigilant in order to avoid falling prey to the artists of confidence and bull.

Skepticism vs Mistrust

It bears repeating that *skepticism and mistrust* are not the same. Skepticism is a healthy point of view among those who seek to verify (when possible) an unknown. Mistrust, on the other hand, is quick to dismiss the truth. It's a subtle difference that's worth remembering when dealing with conspiracy theorists. In the field of medicine, we encounter mistrust in patients and caregivers alike. They test our patience at every turn. Other character flaws include pathologic liars, lazy deadbeats, the irresponsible, habitually late or absent, angry, violent, passive-aggressive, borderline, manipulative, willfully ignorant, self-destructive, and that's just before noon.

How to cope with these character flaws is easier when you apply stoic virtue and remain consistent in your approach. That is, being kind and patient will never get you in trouble. If you encounter someone with a personality disorder such as a borderline personality or a malignant narcissist, you probably shouldn't try too hard to fix it, because you won't. Be thoughtful and provide quality care, and when you're finished, there's another patient waiting in the next room.

"A healthy mind should be prepared for anything."

-Marcus Aurelius

Quotidian Philosophy

The word *quotidian* is derived from the Latin *quotidie* or *daily occurrence,* and *Quotidian Philosophy (QP)* draws our attention to the recurring paroxysms of daily life and the wisdom acquired from it. The refrain of QP—*on again, off again*—occurs in nature. It is evident in our health, our perceptions, and our moods. *On again, off again* is not pathologic or manic or cyclothymic; rather, it reflects the normal oscillations around us and within us, the diurnal variations, circadian rhythms, and other naturally occurring phenomena that come and go. These fluctuations appear random on the surface but are actually predictable, like the Old Faithful Geyser, and those who can recognize this pattern benefit most. It's a paradox that brings comfort to a bad situation (always darkest before the dawn) and helps to buffer the extremes. It makes sense whether you're on top of the world or if everything seems to be going wrong. It helps us remain grounded during the best of times, and attenuates the bad.

An experienced baseball player uses the phrase "staying within myself" to demonstrate this kind of equanimity. One doesn't allow the highs to get too high or the lows to get to low, and batting .300 is great but it also means one will fail to get a hit 70% of the time. If a team wins only 6 out of every 10 games it will likely end up in first place. This sentiment underscores the pendulum that propels a full, rewarding life.

It's a reminder that good times are best appreciated in real time, because the pendulum will continue to swing back and forth until it stops. Nothing in life is certain, except that it will someday end. In the field of medicine this is absolute.

Once again, it is easier to change the things you *do* than who you *are*. You can modify *behavior* such as overeating, smoking, and so forth—we make adjustments all the time—but character and other inherent tendencies are less flexible. You can change the things you *do* more easily than change who you *are*. You can successfully curtail a few bad habits such as gambling or speeding, but these marginal triumphs will not change the fact that you have an impulsive nature. You can temporarily say no to drugs or booze, but the ongoing temptation reflects your addiction. You hear the words of a friend who's trying to help you, but you will not listen until you are ready to help yourself. In a nutshell, that's what the quotidian model is about, the oscillations around us and within us that govern our behavior.

Put differently, if our imperfections are meant to challenge us in some way, the choice basically comes down to two things: acceptance or change. What happens to those who dedicate themselves to self-improvement? It seems like a worthy cause, but the goal itself is a potential trap—a hidden trap that we set for ourselves—and the premise (that we're not good enough) is a set up for despair. That said, if we can accept the flaws of our loved ones, we should be equally accepting of ourselves.

Perhaps there is a compromise to be found by *accepting the things we cannot change*. Any twelve-stepper can tell you that. Alcoholics challenge themselves to remain sober with the wherewithal to get through another day. They help each other by meeting regularly to reinforce the need to change. What are the things that are difficult to change? Character, integrity, wayward impulses, the behavior of *others*—they're all variables that affect our lives and set the stage for a good day or a bad one. Perhaps the struggle boils down to finding more good moments than bad ones, more good days than bad ones, and we do have some control over that.

Stoic Virtue

The four stoic virtues are *justice, temperance* (moderation), *courage,* and *wisdom.* Interestingly, kindness is not listed as one of the big four, although prominent Stoics of the past including Seneca, Epictetus, and Marcus Aurelius made ample references to the importance of *kindness* in their writings. Indeed, the four stoic virtues indirectly pertain to kindness in one way or another, just as fairness, honesty, and empathy do.

Stoicism emerged in Greece around 300 BC around 200 years after the introduction of Buddhism in Asia. Both philosophies are similar in nature valuing inner discipline, virtue, and mindfulness while de-emphasizing transient material goods or vanity. In terms of health, the Stoics promoted exercise and fitness but without undue excess or pride. Two well-known Stoics (Seneca and Musonius) were known to be vegetarians, although nothing in Stoic doctrine forbids eating meat. The placement of these factoids in a book about kindness in healthcare is hardly meant to be comprehensive; my purpose is simply to fold together the principles of virtue and patient care in an effort to move the conversation forward.

At one time or another, adherents of Stoic values have included Thomas Jefferson, and modern thought leaders such as Bill Gates, Warren Buffet, Jack Dorsey, Arianna Huffington, General James Mattis, Cory Booker, Jeff Bazos, and many more. That's not to say these notable people are without flaws or should be held to a higher standard. They would be among the first to tell you that we should only hold *ourselves* to a higher standard. In other words, let us be tolerant of others and strict with ourselves.

The ancient Stoics believed that you were either virtuous or you were not. If you were not virtuous, then by definition you were driven by vice (or *vicious*)—which is to say that, by today's standards, we are all vicious. It's like the Christian maxim suggesting that we are all sinners, a humble viewpoint that serves to unburden our collective souls. In fairness, virtue and vice are matters of degree, like shades of gray or levels of strength, though the writings of the early Stoics and Buddhists suggested that they were less flexible in such matters.

They believed that humans, like other carnivores, are a predatory species that would benefit from self-examination. Any random viewing of the evening news would support this assumption. We declare ourselves virtuous when the situation calls for it, such as inviting a frail senior to step in front of the line at the supermarket, not only because it's the right thing to do, but because it feels good, and we like to feel good.

The *four pillars of kindness* (compassion, empathy, sympathy, and forgiveness) are character traits that offset difficult circumstances and despair. Likewise, the mantra of *virtue* states that *"No man or woman can be moral unless they strive for the benefit of all humanity"* which sounds rather lofty, but the Stoics claimed there is no *degree* of virtue, and therefore no *degree* of vice—you are either one or the other— virtuous or vicious. Some would declare this to be a harsh viewpoint since the vast majority of people reside at the center of this bell-curve; only the sinners and saints inhabit the polar extremes.

If we examine ourselves this way, what do we learn? Humility. Neither sinner nor saint, and that's okay. First do no harm. Try to be kind.

Sense of perspective

For any given situation, a sense of perspective can color one's point of view. Perspectives change depending on the mood of the moment and thereby affect one's opinion or behavior. For example, it has been observed that one's reaction to disappointment (frustration, exasperation, despair) depends less on the news than the person hearing it. Some people crumble at the slightest mishap while others demonstrate composure no matter what. This distinction is at the core of Stoic philosophy.

How to remain composed in a stressful environment requires maturity and experience, and the path forward is not necessarily complicated even for those who have struggled with such things. A sober perspective is to keep *expectations* realistic and adjust them if necessary. We do this all the time in the practice of medicine. For example, when a diagnosis is made and the outlook is grim, a revised goal might be the reduction of suffering. This kind of emotional *reset* doesn't change the outcome but it provides a realistic outlook with less heartache. It's all a matter of perspective.

Personality matters

Any personality type can step up to comfort the sick; some are more effective than others, but no matter who they are, or who they *think* they are, they can help a patient in need. That's because kindness transcends personality; despite everything we've learned about human nature, we are often wrong about the presumption of one's kindness.

The word *personality* is derived from the Latin *persona* or *mask*, which is a hint that people tend to portray themselves differently in one situation or another. It's a game that is played in life, on social media and elsewhere, intentionally or unwittingly. For example, a friendly co-worker may appear happy on the surface because she smiles easily, though she struggles inwardly and carries a terrible burden—or an unsmiling man with a gruff exterior may be misperceived as *unkind* by those who are unaware that he rescues stray dogs and gives generously to charity. So, who are they, really?

We hear the refrain *just be yourself* during trying times of stress or indecision, such as a job interview or the first day of work, but what does that mean? The answer is not complicated. Since no two persons are the same, the best person in any situation—the one that we should always strive to be—is *kind*. And it is worth the effort. Kindness is a *choice* that is difficult for some, easier for others, and the results are generally worthwhile.

"No matter what anyone says or does, my task is to be good."

-Marcus Aurelius

Dealing with hate

It seems that kindness and hate exist in a virtual tug of war. On one side are those who are basically good and want to do good, while the other side is yanked in the opposite direction by a hostile few who can ruin the party for all. And it doesn't take many, sometimes just a single damaged individual with a destructive agenda. So, we protect ourselves and our loved ones while doing our best to help others, and we begin to see that we're all in this together.

Some people who cause harm to others may actually think of themselves as kind. Most of them have a history of personal trauma, which does not excuse bad behavior—they may find refuge in thoughts of hostility, which is understandable if the sentiments are fleeting and no harm is done—but when hostility spills over to affect the lives of others, we have a problem.

There are also kind people who have suffered trauma but carry on nonetheless. We may not know who they are but we see them every day. They put out the fires. They plant trees. They feed the hungry and care for the sick. They make art and music, write romance novels and comic strips, root for teams, spend time with family and friends, cook and clean, and *first do no harm*.

That's a lot of people doing good. The cumulative effect of doing *good* creates an environment of hope. It may sound saccharine but there is more *good* in the world than *bad*, more love than hate, even if it feels like the opposite is true. It may seem on the evening news that the bad guys winning, but they are not. And they never will. In all of mankind's history the haters had their day until they were laid to rest.

Hate has always been around like cancer and heart attacks and criminals who prey upon victims—but then new babies are born and children grow up to be nurses and teachers and mothers who clean up the mess and make things better again. One person at a time moves the needle a tiny fraction, like an ant in a giant colony whose role may seem miniscule but is essential for survival. That's what kindness in healthcare is all about.

Forgiveness

In an ideal world forgiveness is a win-win for everyone. But it's complicated. I remember watching footage of the tragic Charleston, SC shooting in which a young white man slaughtered nine church members in a race-motivated ambush in the basement of their church. In the days that followed I recall seeing the heart-wrenching strain with which the surviving family members "forgave" the murderer.

My heart went out to those nice people, the grief-stricken mourners who reached deep inside to utter words of forgiveness even though it appeared they weren't quite ready to forgive. The pain of loss, still raw in their faces as the cameras rolled, was evident. "I forgive you" they each proclaimed in succession through their tears.

Why did they forgive him? There are several reasons. First, the Savior in their scripture was the model of forgiveness, and they were obliged to follow His teachings. Second, by forgiving the murderer, they were able to assume a bit of control over the situation, and third, to deprive him of the satisfaction he might have otherwise claimed. No doubt, to simply move on after a tragedy like that is impossible. There is no correct way to rectify the situation, but there are lots of wrong ways to do it. I give the mourning family members credit for trying. There are too many legacies of hate and revenge in the world. It had to stop somewhere.

Why is this relevant to a book about kindness in medicine? Because tragedies occur all the time in medicine, and forgiveness is in short supply. People get mad at the world—mad at God or their spouse or the government or their doctor or nurse. We need to be prepared for untoward behavior in the wake of tragedy, whether it is anger directed at a staff member, criticism of a provider, or frustration by patients or family members in the aftermath of a poor medical outcome. There is no need to condone harassment, intimidation, or threatening behavior, but to make every effort to remain calm and understanding when emotions run high.

Forgiveness is a two-way street, and caregivers must take the lead by setting a good example. That means being forgiving to others as we would want them to be to us, not only to clerical staff and students who make occasional mistakes, but to patients, transporters, runners, janitorial staff, and so on. Once a brief, private, thoughtful discussion is shared, letting them off-the-hook for an unintentional error is good practice.

Getting older

Quotidian Philosophy refers to the illusion of change—which is not to say that change in ourselves doesn't occur, but if it happens at all it occurs too slowly to notice—like watching the grass grow. One example is the process of getting older. For some aging is a wonderful thing, a chance to move forward in life and experience new memories; for others it's a constant threat, a cloud that ominously hovers.

At the end of life, the human body will either wither and decompose or be incinerated, and none of it goes to waste. Basic conservation of energy demands that flesh and bone will decay gradually, or it will be quickly cremated, and in either situation it will go back to the well of energy and molecules that will be absorbed by countless bacteria and wild birds, nourish crops and become the food we eat, the clothes we wear, or the particles we breathe every day. In this way we are all immortal. It's not quite like heaven, but it's really okay. The point is, there is no need to be afraid.

Getting older has benefits, such as attaining wisdom and experience, enjoying time to relax and reflect on a life well lived—but it also means the accumulation of failures, physical limitations, lost opportunities, and a path toward an uncertain end. Happily, the *acceptance* of life's palindromes makes the struggle less burdensome. It's a point of view that becomes evident with age, a reminder to embrace the passage of time, to let go of material needs and ego-driven conquests, and enjoy the moment. That is what wisdom and kindness are all about.

Why complain?

At the core of each complaint is a sense of hardship that is sometimes justifiable, although in most cases *complaining* has *less* to do with the complaint than the *complainer.* It begs the question, when is it okay to complain?

Surely there are minor annoyances that affect all of us—a cancelled flight, a flat tire—which are manageable, yet we tend to complain anyway. At the far end of the spectrum are the tragedies that randomly befall victims, such as violent crime, terminal cancer, natural disasters, and other serious hardships, with a wide berth to complain, if desired. Certain individuals artfully deal with minor setbacks in real time and rarely complain; others shrug them off but complain nonetheless, and then there are those who catastrophize everything.

I raise the question because caregivers are squarely in the business of listening to complaints. Within the scope of a few minutes, we might encounter a privileged patient who complains bitterly about minor elbow discomfort because it interferes with five hours of golf, while in the next exam room a patient with terminal cancer carries on quietly and feels thankful for another day. Their circumstances are different as their thresholds to complain, but we instinctively set aside judgment. Rather, we give each patient what they need.

One may ask, do unhappy people complain more? The answer is yes. Is it a rich versus poor thing? Sometimes, although once a person has escaped the ranks of poverty and secures the essentials of food and shelter, money makes less difference than we might think. In fact, it's been observed that the happiest people on earth are not necessarily the wealthiest. Happiness is experienced by those who cultivate friendships, find a sense of purpose, enjoy family ties and a sense of community. In America, as in other highly industrialized nations, greater wealth does not guarantee happiness. Too often, people run up credit cards or find themselves beholden to a huge mortgage or the demands of an unsatisfying job, yet how often people do exactly that.

I've seen the deteriorating health of those who dislike their jobs or work too much and cannot find a moment to rest. They eventually learn that the human body has its limits—cardiovascular, metabolic, immune, mental health—and even a healthy body will shut down if you abuse it.

Money issues aside, it has also been observed that intelligence and happiness do not correlate. There is little argument that it's good to be smart. But not always. And not too smart. For example, in matters of happiness, those of average intelligence are more likely to find fun and friendship among others of a similar average IQ whereas highly intelligent people find enjoyment but in different ways and with certain barriers. By nature, the smartest people in the crowd may be predisposed to depression, boredom, and cynicism.

It's an unspoken disadvantage that few discuss candidly. It's difficult for the average person to appreciate the frustration and isolation at either extreme of the intelligence spectrum—the super smart and the less than average—wishing they could connect better with the mainstream. In the grand scheme of things, nobody is shedding tears for smart people, especially the high-income earners given the multitude of benefits they enjoy, but it helps to remember that everyone suffers quietly in some way. With this in mind, we should be kind to all regardless of their rung on the ladder, since we can never be certain of the frustration in their lives.

Ask the exhausted mother of a colicky newborn what would be nice and she would probably tell you *a good night's sleep*. Ask an overworked factory employee and she might say *time off*. Ask a lonely senior and his response might be *some company*. It helps to remember this when simple pleasures come our way.

People *want* things they may never have, and *have* things they will never want. For the average person, meeting the ordinary demands of work to pay bills and raise a family is enough of a reason to complain. People fantasize about the *good life*, free of worry, free to enjoy a moment of peace or simply relax. They plan the long road to freedom (usually financial freedom) by saving and working their entire lives for a future that may never come. Along the way, the job of healthcare providers includes listening to their complaints and helping them stay healthy so they can carry on.

What is Normal?

The definition of *normal* is constantly changing. For example, the results of most blood tests fall within a bell-curve under which 95% are considered normal and the other 5% at either end are flagged as abnormal. Yet for some individuals a presumed abnormality may be *normal for them*: a low mean corpuscular volume is *expected* in one with Thalassemia but in others may raise a red flag of iron deficiency anemia, a sign of blood loss or poor nutrition. A soft heart murmur may be perfectly fine in a patient who's always had it, but if the murmur is suddenly new it could be a problem.

How does the concept of *normal* pertain to kindness? In terms of behavior, *normal* is a reflection of tolerance—*normal* is what society decides it is—and it is constantly changing. For example, at the dawn of television in the early 1950's, married couples were not permitted to be shown (or even implied to be) sleeping in the same bed. The rules of modesty required that spousal beds had to be separated by a night table. Even gestational Lucy Ricardo, whose bed was conveniently near Ricky's, was not permitted to use the word "pregnant." She was "expecting." We look back on these puritanical oddities as woefully outdated, but in 1954 America, these guardrails were considered normal.

There's little doubt that what is *normal* now will not necessarily remain so. Films of baseball games from the 1930's show thousands of men wearing the exact same ridiculous style of straw hat. It begs the question, which of our current norms will someday be looked back upon as folksy or backward? Can anyone really know? The answer may be suspected by those with a keen sense of foresight or intuition, but for most people the future is vague. The great innovators in history stand out as having a unique gift of anticipation. Henry Ford didn't invent the car but he foresaw the merits of mass production. Steve Jobs didn't invent the cell phone or the computer, but he envisioned the needs and desires of the masses—the new normal.

The notion of *normal* varies from culture to culture, and *change*, if any, occurs slowly. Advances in women's rights, racial tolerance, gender identity, and so on have been a roller coaster ride with opinions all over the place, and many who have suffered. Likewise, in medicine, in addition to the racial and gender biases that remain problematic, medical advice for patients has evolved over the centuries. If you crack open any medical textbook written over 100 years ago, you'll find that most of the information (with the exception of anatomy) is incorrect, yet we've managed to survive. The point is that we should never be so arrogant to think we know everything. Whatever is considered normal today may change over time. It's a state of mind that's helpful when listening to those whose opinions may differ from yours.

This brings us to the topic of conflicting beliefs, intolerance, and the struggle to coexist. From Romeo and Juliet to West Side Story, there have been examples of relationships that thrive and endure when people of goodwill want them to, or fail when goodwill is the target of disruption. Unfortunately, it doesn't take much to spoil the party. In healthcare, an initial patient encounter, like any new relationship, is a sensitive one. For this reason, we strive for good behavior and minimize any outside influences such as politics, religion, or extreme points of view that can disrupt an early encounter. In other words, keep the initial discussion light and save the heavy stuff for another day.

"Self-control, goodwill to others, and every similar virtue... will make you more gentle to all."

-Marcus Aurelius

Faith

Defining *faith* is like trying to define *love*. Sometimes mere words are better left unspoken or the magic disappears. Similarly, reducing faith to conventional language is complicated, and perhaps we shouldn't try. If a virtuous man proclaims that a certain prophet is his savior, or that the only path to paradise is by accepting the scripture of a specific book, who really benefits by suggesting otherwise? If one finds comfort in religious belief, why offer a sterile analysis or a rebuttal?

Unlike the practice of medicine, faith is a source of well-being that transcends belief; it is highly personal and affects each individual differently. There are no two Christians who believe exactly the same thing, and the same can be said for any two Muslims, Jews or atheists. Faith is what we *allow* ourselves to believe.

Conversely, medical decisions by healthcare professionals are rarely based on faith alone. Doctors and nurses are asked to rely on evidence-based data; they are trained to question the validity of isolated testimonials, observations, and opinions in the absence of proof. They understand there is plenty of room for prayer in the hearts and minds of those who deliver healthcare, as long as faith is not the sole arbiter of medical decisions.

Our medical office represents an assortment of religious beliefs that range from non-believer to evangelical, and a similarly diverse collection of interns, residents and medical students who arrive from every corner of the globe to participate in elective rotations; they work alongside doctors, PA's, nurses, and other team members whose differing stances in politics and religion create no discernable tension, because our attention to the patients comes first.

Each healthcare professional is a link in a chain that is built to serve others. We are interdependent in this way: there is no provider without patients, no illness without health, and nothing in the doctrine of any religion that conflicts with being a good humanitarian. Ours is a voice that says "do unto others" and "love thy neighbor" as stated in the scripture. The freedom to believe in a divine presence (or not) is valued and accepted by caregivers, as long as no harm is done. We accept the religious views of our colleagues even when we have differing points of view. What we do have in common is *each other.* We share birthday celebrations, donations to charity events, lunch in the lounge, devotion to our patients and each other. It's an agenda that transcends religion, race, political affiliation, and more. It fills our hearts and it sustains us. Toward that end, we are all humanitarians.

"My religion is simple—my religion is kindness"

-Dalai Lama

When you consider the negatives that are so pervasive in society— poverty, greed, illness, violence, tragedy, and despair—a durable faith in humanity recognizes that most people are basically good, and life is worth living. It's an existential worldview that the time we share on earth is precious. I've comforted people at their most vulnerable and seen others at their bravest, and within that spectrum is the plain truth that our responses to life's adversities vary considerably. Such is the human condition. If a patient believes that a higher power is guiding my clinical decisions, that's fine with me.

Ultimately, faith comes in countless forms, including the practice of religion. Teammates can have faith in each other; family members and co-workers as well. The priority of religion in one's life and the interpretations of religion are infinitely varied. For example, one soldier might place God before country, while another may place family above all other concerns. Who's to say which is right? Those who claim to have all the answers would find themselves on shaky ground.

Think about it, what kind of argument (and we've heard them all) would change your mind about religion? Or the abortion issue? Or the right to bear arms? The intricacies of belief are so deeply rooted and varied in the minds of otherwise well-meaning people that one should never presume to know what is certain, or insist on what matters most to another. It goes to the true meaning of kindness to tolerate the differing views of patients and colleagues, for their sake and our own.

State of Grace

Grace is a virtue expressed in our thoughts, attitudes, and behavior. Good deeds and charity, for example, are time-tested vehicles for grace. Doing good does not require an emotional overhaul or an epiphany, just an opportunity.

It's been said, "If you are more fortunate than others, build a longer table, not a taller fence." But how many people actually subscribe to this? The sentiment is more common in theory than practice. Ultimately, grace is about *gratitude, giving,* and *forgiving.*

"A candle sacrifices nothing by lighting another..."

Giving is the easiest thing in the world, except when it's not. For example, I've regularly donated money to Doctors-Without-Borders, but I've never actually served in a war-torn region. For one reason or another, my capacity for altruism and bravery have not quite reached that level. And that's too bad for me, since providing care in a distant place to people in desperate need might have been the experience of a lifetime. Suffice to say that a good deed is just a step away from us all. The hardest part is just beginning.

In some cases, *giving* is easier than *forgiving*. How withholding we can be to spare a few precious words. Yet we do this all the time. Our charitable instincts kick in for those in need, our protective instincts surface for those in trouble, yet too often the simplest words of forgiveness are stubbornly withheld from those who need to hear them most. It's a gift that is readily available: a call on the phone, a thoughtful letter. What is the force that makes forgiveness—or an apology—so challenging when it's among the easiest tasks? Perhaps the answer lies in simple grace. Like kindness, it's a matter of practice.

ACKNOWLEDGEMENTS:

I am grateful to friends, patients, and colleagues whose guidance, expertise, and kindness have contributed to the pages of *Let Me Help*, including Alla Rudinskaya, Vadim Tikhomirov, Svetlana Tikhomirova, Vicki Blumberg, Ginger Hannon, Bill Delaney, Davd Weinshel, JoAnn Maroto-Soltis, Evanne Orlean, Janaka Periyapperruma, John Stratidis, Beth Aaronson, Majid Sadigh, Cortney Davis, Sydney Page, Jen Heckmann, Jessica Edwards Palmieri, Tiffany Brett, Samantha Lopez McKinney, Chelsea LaBow Murphy, Kimberly Ofoegbu, Essie Daniels, Crystal Jaquez, Vanessa Alves, Connie Reinders, Isabel Ramos-DeSousa, Linda Wheeler, Barbara Eisinger, Dillan Suggs, Joan Anderson, Joan Fiore, Shannon Rajotte, Veronica Duarte James, CJ Francis, Osra Christie, Heather Weinbrum, Deborah Burns, Anita Adzima, Janice Murner, Sal Sena, Rick Pope, Mike Spiegel, Marcie Wolinsky, Joyce Reyes Thomas, Mohamed Mohamed, Karan Chawdhary, Alison Jakubek, Lynn Cohen, Lisa Kamas, Cathy Grellet, Gloria Assad, Gloria Weinshel, Ed Volpintesta, Joe Belskey, Marvin Prince, John Pezzimenti, David Copen, Jon Alexander, John Burris, John Lunt, Marty Abrams, Howard Garfinkel, Winston Shih, Jan Mashman, Lauren Balsanello Pueraro, Jim Kenny, Leo Blachar, Jeff Dreznick, Noel Robin, Bob Gifford, Joe Craft, John Hardin, Steve Malawista, Leo Cooney, Gary Dreiblatt, Pyser Edelsack, and Neil DeGrasse Tyson.

ABOUT THE AUTHOR

*D*avid Trock has written in several genres including medical journals, book chapters, non-fiction books "Healing Fibromyalgia" and "Let Me Help," and a humanist murder mystery titled, "A Religion Called Love." He grew up in Brooklyn, NY and lives in Connecticut with his wife, Elise.

SYNOPSIS:

The Best Decisions Begin With Kindness.

In an era of busy doctors, virtual visits, electronic records, and complicated insurance, patients are feeling frustrated. *Let Me Help* is a reminder that ***patient satisfaction*** begins with kindness and is achievable by following a few simple principles.

The inspiring words of *Let Me Help* include patient narratives, advice for young caregivers, champions of healthcare, and stirring accounts depicted by the author. Readers of *Let Me Help* will quickly recognize the keys to patient satisfaction, better clinical results, and the rewards of a career in healthcare.

Made in United States
Orlando, FL
13 December 2023

40827222R00125